A MONUMENT TO GOOD INTENTIONS

The Story of the
Maryland Penitentiary, 1804 – 1995

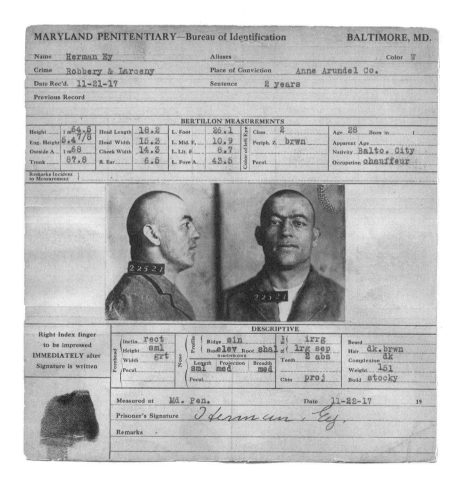

MARYLAND PENITENTIARY—Bureau of Identification   BALTIMORE, MD.

Name	Herman Ey	Aliases	Color W
Crime	Robbery & Larceny	Place of Conviction	Anne Arundel Co.
Date Rec'd.	11-21-17	Sentence	2 years
Previous Record			

BERTILLON MEASUREMENTS

Height	1 m 64.5	Head Length	18.2	L. Foot	26.1	Class 2	Age 28 Born in 1
Eng. Height	5.4 7/8	Head Width	15.2	L. Mid. F.	10.9	Periph. Z. brwn	Apparent Age
Outside A	1 m 68	Cheek Width	14.3	L. Lit. F.	8.7		Nativity Balto. City
Trunk	87.8	R. Ear	6.5	L. Fore A.	43.5	Pecul.	Occupation chauffeur

Remarks Incident to Measurement

DESCRIPTIVE

Right Index finger to be impressed IMMEDIATELY after Signature is written

Inclin. rect	Ridge sin	irrg
Height sml	Base elev Root shal	lrg sep
Width grt	DIMENSIONS	2 abs
Pecul.	Length sml Projection med Breadth med	Chin proj
	Pecul.	

Beard	
Hair dk. brwn	
Complexion dk	
Weight 151	
Build stocky	

Measured at   Md. Pen.   Date 11-22-17   19

Prisoner's Signature   Herman Ey

Remarks

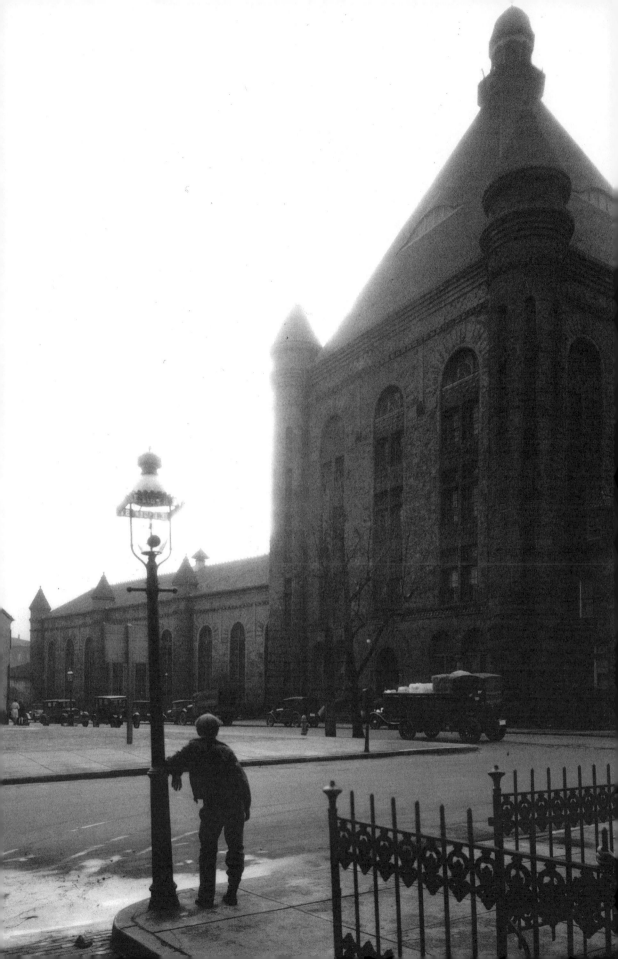

A
MONUMENT
TO GOOD
INTENTIONS

The Story of the Maryland Penitentiary
1804 – 1995

WALLACE SHUGG

MARYLAND HISTORICAL SOCIETY

Baltimore, Maryland

MARYLAND HISTORICAL SOCIETY

201 West Monument Street

Baltimore, Maryland 21201

LIBRARY OF CONGRESS CATALOGING-IN-PUBLICATION DATA

Shugg, Wallace, 1929-
   A monument to good intentions: the story of the Maryland Peniten-
tiary, 1804-1995 / Wallace Shugg.
      p. cm.
   Includes bibliographical references and index.
   ISBN 0-938420-91-7 (cloth : alk. paper) – ISBN 0-938420-92-5 (pbk. :
alk. paper)
      1. Maryland Penitentiary—History.   2. Prisons—Maryland—
History.   I. Title:
Story of the Maryland Penitentiary, 1804-1995.   II. Title.

HV9475.M32 M378 2000
365'.97526—dc21   99-053286

Manufactured in the United States of America
The paper used in this publication meets the minimum
requirements of the American National Standard for Information Sciences
Permanence of Paper for Printed Library Materials ANSI Z39.48-1984.

To Captain Robert Lee Burrell

Contents

Preface

Thanks to American prison films, the word "penitentiary" today suggests to many people a warehouse of steel cellblocks designed with the worst intentions to grind down the souls of criminals. But unlike the older word "prison," with its basic meaning of simple confinement behind stone walls and iron bars, "penitentiary" originated as a quasi-religious term, suggesting a monastic environment intended to reform souls. It was coined by prison reformers in the 1770s[1] and first used by the English philosopher Jeremy Bentham in 1776, according to the *Oxford English Dictionary*.

The penitentiary concept arose in England during the Age of Enlightenment and was viewed by its supporters as an improvement over the usual treatment of criminals.[2] At the time, minor offenders, such as vagrants and prostitutes, were summarily dealt with by corporal punishment: the stocks, pillory, whipping post, or branding iron. Relatively few criminals were punished by long-term imprisonment. Prisons and jails were mainly for the temporary detention of debtors or more serious offenders awaiting trial or execution, or transportation under terms of servitude to the American colonies. The most infamous of the London prisons, Old Newgate, typified the haphazard penal conditions of the time. Never planned as a prison, it was a noisy, crowded stone labyrinth in which well-to-do offenders paid the jailer extortionate fees for comfortable lodgings in private apartments, while the less fortunate were herded together in common wards, without regard to age, sex, or criminal offense and where dirt, disease, idleness, gambling, drinking, and fornication prevailed.[3] This vicious atmosphere was hardly conducive to

---

1. John B. Bender, *Imagining the Penitentiary: Fictions and the Architecture of Mind in Eighteenth-Century England* (Chicago: University of Chicago Press, 1987), p. 208.

2. This sketch of the rise of the penitentiary idea is drawn from Bender, *Imagining the Penitentiary*, pp.13–29, Blake McKelvey, *American Prisons: A History of Good Intentions* (Montclair, N.J.: Patterson Smith, 1977), pp. 1–3, Harry E. Barnes and Negley Teeters, *New Horizons in Criminology*, 3rd ed. (Englewood Cliffs, N.J.: Prentice-Hall, 1959), pp. 328–29, and especially Robin Evans, *The Fabrication of Virtue: English Prison Architecture, 1750–1840* (Cambridge: Cambridge University Press, 1982), pp. 47–93.

3. Conditions at Newgate are thoroughly described in Evans, *Fabrication of Virtue*, pp. 19, 21, 26, 28, 32, 34–40.

the reformation of criminals, a point frequently emphasized by prison reformers when they quoted St. Paul (I Corinthians 15:33): "evil communication corrupts."

In the mid-1770s, the English prison reformer John Howard inspected jails and workhouses in England and on the Continent and published his findings in a highly influential work, *The State of the Prisons in England and Wales* (1777). The movement led by this crusader resulted in the Penitentiary Act of 1779, which called for the construction of "penitentiary houses" throughout the realm. The act abolished fees and aimed at reforming criminals "by sobriety, by cleanliness and medical assistance, by a regular series of labour, by solitary confinement during intervals of work . . . to inure them to the habits of industry, to guard them from pernicious company."[4] Although some jails sought to comply with the provisions of the Penitentiary Act,[5] no penitentiary houses were erected in England for a variety of reasons—lack of funds, debate over the choice of a site for the first penitentiary, and the opening up of Australia for the transportation of large numbers of convicts. But the penitentiary idea traveled across the Atlantic to the New World, where it was taken up by those interested in prison reform. The first penitentiaries were actually constructed on American soil.

Prison reforms in the American colonies had been initiated by the Quakers. As early as 1682, the Quaker proprietor William Penn brought with him a new legal corpus, the "Great Law," to his newly founded Province of Pennsylvania. It included the original Quaker criminal code. Among other things, instead of the corporal punishment for criminals called for by the harsh code that prevailed in England, it prescribed imprisonment at hard labor in houses of correction as a punishment for most major offenders and in a later supplement reduced the number of capital crimes to one: premeditated murder. This more humane Quaker code provided the basis for the treatment of criminals in the province until Penn's death in 1718, when it was replaced by the "sanguinary laws" of the mother country, listing thirteen capital offenses. The practice of whipping, branding, and mutilation had meanwhile crept into the province from other colonies. These severe penalties remained in force until the post-revolutionary revision of the Pennsylvania criminal code in 1786.[6]

The revised penal code was less draconian, inasmuch as it substituted sentences at hard labor for capital punishment for all but two major offenses. But one result was the practice of sending convicts out in wheelbarrow gangs to work on

---

4. Barnes and Teeters, *New Horizons in Criminology,* pp. 329–35.

5. One of them, erected at Wymondham in Norfolk under the management of Thomas Beevor, was to provide a pattern for those who established the first American penitentiary. See McKelvey, *American Prisons,* p. 14, and Evans, *Fabrication of Virtue,* p. 73.

6. Barnes and Teeters, *New Horizons in Criminology,* pp. 325–27, and McKelvey, *American Prisons,* p. 25.

public roads and in city streets.[7] The security measures deemed necessary produced a disturbing spectacle. Convicts, according to an early historian, were

> encumbered with iron collars and chains, to which bomb-shells were attached, to be dragged along while they performed their degrading service, under the eyes of keepers armed with swords, blunderbusses, and other weapons of destruction. These measures begot in the minds of the criminals and those who witnessed them, disrespect for the laws executed with such cruelty.[8]

On March 9, 1787, a Quaker physician, Benjamin Rush, delivered an address at the home of Benjamin Franklin, *An Enquiry into the Effects of Public Punishments Upon Criminals and Upon Society* (1787). Among other things, Dr. Rush argued that "all public punishments tend to make bad men worse, and to increase crimes" by destroying "the sense of shame" and breeding in them "a spirit of revenge." He urged that "a house of repentance" be erected for the private punishment of criminals, inside of which they would be subjected to solitude, silence, religious instruction and labor "profitable to the State."[9]

On May 8, 1787 a group of Quakers and others who shared Dr. Rush's views regarding the treatment of criminals formed the Philadelphia Society for Alleviating the Miseries of Public Prisons. In 1790 another reform law was passed, incorporating suggestions made by the new society. As a result, the "wheelbarrow men" were taken off the streets, and the yard of the Walnut Street Jail in Philadelphia was provided with facilities for the solitary confinement of "the more hardened offenders" and a work program for prisoners, making it—according to Negley K. Teeters—the first penitentiary in the world.[10] The initial success of this penitentiary experiment during the years 1790–1799 ("the heydey of the Walnut Street Jail") gained the attention of other eastern states, including Maryland, which in 1804 set about imitating the example of the Philadelphia reformers.[11]

The Maryland Penitentiary is now the oldest operating penitentiary in the world.[12] The only remnant of its original structures (1811) visible to the passerby

---

7. McKelvey, *American Prisons*, p. 7.

8. Roberts Vaux, *Notices of the Original and Successive Efforts to Improve the Discipline of the Prison at Philadelphia and to Reform the Criminal Code of Pennsylvania: with a few observations on the penitentiary system* (Philadelphia: Kimber and Sharpless, 1826), pp. 21–22.

9. Rush, *An Enquiry,* pp. 4, 12, 13. In urging the provision of a block of solitary cells, Dr. Rush had in mind the example set by the recently constructed county jail in Norfolk, England, which had sought to comply with the reform proposals of John Howard (McKelvey, *American Prisons,* p. 8).

10. Negley K. Teeters, *The Cradle of the Penitentiary: The Walnut Street Jail at Philadelphia, 1773–1835* (Philadelphia, 1955), pp. 17–19, 30, 39–40, 61.

11. Vaux, *Notices,* pp. 31, 34. Maryland's penitentiary was the fifth (completed 1811), after New York (1796), Virginia (1800), Massachusetts (1804), and Vermont (1808). See Donald Cressey's introduction to Francis C. Gray, *Prison Discipline in America* [London, 1848] (repr. Montclair, N.J.: Patterson Smith, 1973), p. vi.

12. Interview, August 19, 1987, with Professor Peter P. Lejins, former Director of the Institute of

today is the twenty-foot-high stone wall running along the north side of Madison Street between the City Jail yard and Forrest Street. On the corner one block northeast stands the castle-like granite administration building (1899), with its cavernous west wing extending along Eager Street. Within its 5½ acre plot over the past 185 years, numerous other buildings of varied size, shape, and purpose have come and gone: a time-lapse film—say, a frame shot every week—would yield the spectacle of dormitories, stables, sheds, workshops and other outbuildings of wood or masonry rising from the ground, flourishing for a period, perhaps acquiring an additional story or wing, and then vanishing by means of fire, crowbar or wrecker's ball, to be replaced by some newer structure. During its most recent period of growth, the penitentiary has spilled over its walls into the surrounding neighborhood with the construction of such satellites as the Reception-Diagnostic & Classification Center (1981) at the corner of Madison and Greenmount Streets and the Maryland Correctional Adjustment Center or "Supermax" (1989), diagonally across Madison Street and opposite the City Jail.

Because it is a complex patchwork of the old and the new, the Maryland Penitentiary is a difficult subject for a history, especially for its early years. Few illustrations of it exist before the twentieth century, and so the lineaments of some of its vanished buildings must be inferred from sketchy contemporary descriptions or imagined from crude drawings on old maps. The surviving administration records, whether in manuscript or print, are scattered throughout the state at various institutions. After 1900 photos of the penitentiary and newspaper articles about it become more numerous but for the most part are not indexed and must be searched out on microfilm. It is perhaps because of these difficulties that no one in this century has published a history of the penitentiary.[13]

This essay aims not at giving an exhaustive history but rather an overall view of the development of this venerable institution. During the penitentiary's long existence, its administrators have almost always responded to the prevailing climate of opinion about what a prison should be architecturally and how prisoners

---

Criminal Justice and Criminology at the University of Maryland, College Park. One must keep in mind the distinction between penitentiaries and prisons—many of the latter were built earlier and a few continue to operate in some form. If the penitentiary reportedly built by Catherine the Great of Russia in the late eighteenth century is still operating, then the Maryland Penitentiary is the oldest continuously operating penitentiary in the *Western* World. The Virginia State Penitentiary in Richmond, the only surviving one older (1800) than Maryland's, was recently phased out, a process completed at the end of 1990 (*Baltimore Sun,* November 25, 1990).

13. Early historical sketches appeared in *Testimony Taken Before the Joint Committee of the Legislature on the Penitentiary* (Annapolis, 1837), pp. 8–13; the appendix of the annual *Board of Directors Report* (1881), pp. 33–95; J. Thomas Scharf's *History of Baltimore City and County* (1881), pp. 202–5; and the *Report of the Maryland Penitentiary Penal Commission* (1913), Appendix B. Marvin Gettleman's "The Maryland Penitentiary in the Age of Tocqueville, 1828–1842," *Maryland Historical Magazine,* 56 (1961): 269–90, deals with that period only.

should be treated. And so this essay should also provide the reader with a useful survey of the changing fashions in prison architecture and penology in this country for the past 185 years—"a history of good intentions," to borrow an apt phrase.[14] The bibliography and appendices should help those who wish to pursue in detail certain aspects of the penitentiary's complex history.

Chapter one, "The Early Years, 1804–1836," describes the construction of its original buildings with dungeon-like cells and its struggle to support itself by prison labor in the pre-industrial age. Chapter two, "The Investigation of 1837," tells how the existence of the young institution was threatened by political conflict both outside and inside its walls. Chapter three, "New Ways in Penology," covers the next half century, during which time the penitentiary experimented with innovative practices from other prisons or fresh theories and ideas from prison reformers. Chapter four, "The Rise and Fall of Warden John F. Weyler, 1888–1920," describes the prison's evolution into a modern penitentiary with steel cellblocks but with a harshly efficient administration that had to give way to more progressive penal methods. Chapter five, "Reform Methods on Trial, 1920–1960," tells how these methods were tempered and followed by a long and stable administration. Chapter six, "The Years of Political Turmoil, 1960–1980," shows the impact on the penitentiary of the Civil Rights movement, anti-Vietnam War sentiment, and accompanying drug culture. Chapter seven, "Keeping the Lid On, 1981–1995," is about the efforts of prison officials to deal with overcrowding, as a crime-weary public called for tougher sentencing laws and tighter parole policies.

I take pleasure in thanking the American Correctional Association, Enoch Pratt Free Library, Maryland Division of Correction, Maryland Historical Society Library, Maryland State Archives (Hall of Records), Maryland State Law Library, and the Interlibrary Loan Department of the University of Maryland Baltimore County Library. The University of Maryland Baltimore County Graduate School provided generous support in the form of a faculty research grant.

Many people helped with the making of this book. I would like to thank especially Jo Bateman, Audrey Brown, Robert Lee Burrell, Leo Burroughs, Clarence Davis, Alan Eason, Walter Farrier, James Felix, Preston Fitzberger, the late Martin ("Jitterbug Slim") Groves, Svend Hansen, McLindsey Hawkins, Elmanus Herndon, Tom Hollowak, Jeffrey Korman, William Jednorski, Peter Lejins, Harry Loftice, Howard Lyles, Gerald McClellan, David O'Dunne, Francis O'Neill, Theodore Purnell, Barbara D. Rinehimer, Alan Scherr, Sewall Smith, Pamela Sorensen, the late Thomas Tivvis, Harry Traurig, and Wesley Wilson.

---

14. McKelvey, *American Prisons*.

I would also like to thank Warden Eugene Nuth for his support; Andrew Stritch, my eyes and ears inside "the Castle"; and Bernadine Dembeck for a heroic typing job. Only her interest in the penitentiary's history could have sustained her while wading through the thickets and tangles of an untidy manuscript.

In particular I would like to thank publisher Robert I. Cottom, editors Patricia Anderson and Donna Shear, and photographer David Prencipe of the Maryland Historical Society's press, designers Gerard A. Valerio and James F. Brisson, and Ernest L. Scott for making this a better book.

Catonsville, Maryland
March 1999

A Monument to Good Intentions

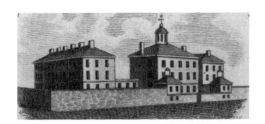

Names	Places of Nativity	Age	Complexion	
Negro Bob	Calvert County	22 years	Black	Sla...
Negro Will	Montgomery Coty	50 years	Yellow	Sla...
Negro Faraway	Anne Arundel Cty	23 years	Black	Sla...
Joseph J. H. Caulk	Delaware	33 years	Dark	
Negro Sam	Anne Arundel Cty	31 years	Black	Slave
Negro James	Montgomery Cty	31 years	Yellow	Slave
Negro Joe	Harford County	24 years	Black	Sla...
Negro Harry	Harford County	20 years	Black	Sla...
Negro Cyrus	Harford County	25 years	Black	Sla...
William Smith	Jamaica	unknown	Black	
James Perry	Baltimore City	23 years	Fair	
James Linton	Sweden	20 years	Dark	
Negro James	St. Marys County	21 years	Black	
Negro Thomas alias James	Virginia	35 years	Black	
Negro Tom	Cecil County	27 years	Black	Slave
Daniel Coker	Caroline County	46 years	Yellow	
Joseph Woodward +	St. Marys County	30 years	Light	
Major Truff	Worcester County	50 years	Black	Slave
Nickl Rice	Harford County	29 years	Black	Slave
Negro Harry	Anne Arundel Cty	21 years	Black	Slave
Jacob Lockler	Frederick County	24 years	Yellow	Slave
Nicholas Queen	St. Marys County	47 years	Black	
Negro George	Frederick County	48 years	Black	Sla...

Chapter One

The Early Years

1804 – 1836

On November 18, 1811, a twenty-two-year-old slave and convicted murderer, "Negro Bob" Butler, became the first inmate to enter the Maryland Penitentiary.[1] Along with fifty other criminals working in wheelbarrow gangs cleaning and repairing the streets and basin of Baltimore Town, he had been offered the chance to serve out his sentence inside the newly constructed penitentiary, away from the public eye. The opening of the prison was reported "with uncommon pleasure" by the weekly *Niles' Register,* which noted the expiration of "the semi-barbarous wheelbarrow-law" and spoke of the first inmates as "privileged."[2]

The penitentiary had been erected by the State of Maryland in response to a widespread antipathy to the spectacle of convicts working on public roads. And in so doing, it had acted with good intentions, as was apparent from the very beginning. At its November session in 1804, the legislature appointed nine commissioners to choose a site for the prison and to propose a plan to the governor; among them were public-spirited men notable for their contributions to the burgeoning port-town.[3] By

---

[1]Born in 1789 in Calvert County, Butler's original sentence of death was commuted to life on October 20, 1803, probably because of his youth. He died on October 24, 1855, at age sixty-six after having served forty-four years. Maryland Penitentiary, Reception Records, #5655, Maryland State Archives.

[2]November 30, 1811.

[3]The commissioners, who served without pay, are listed in *The Acts of Assembly, together with the Governor's proclamation and rules and regulations, respecting the penitentiary of Maryland* (Baltimore, 1819), p. 3, and included

Left: Detail from the first prisoners reception book. The first prisoner to enter the new Maryland State Penitentiary was a slave, "Negro Bob" Butler, convicted of murder in 1803 at the age of fourteen. (Maryland State Archives.)

Overleaf: Warner & Hanna's Plan of the City & Environs of Baltimore, 1801. The new jail, and later the penitentiary, are located just north of Old Town. (Maryland Historical Society).

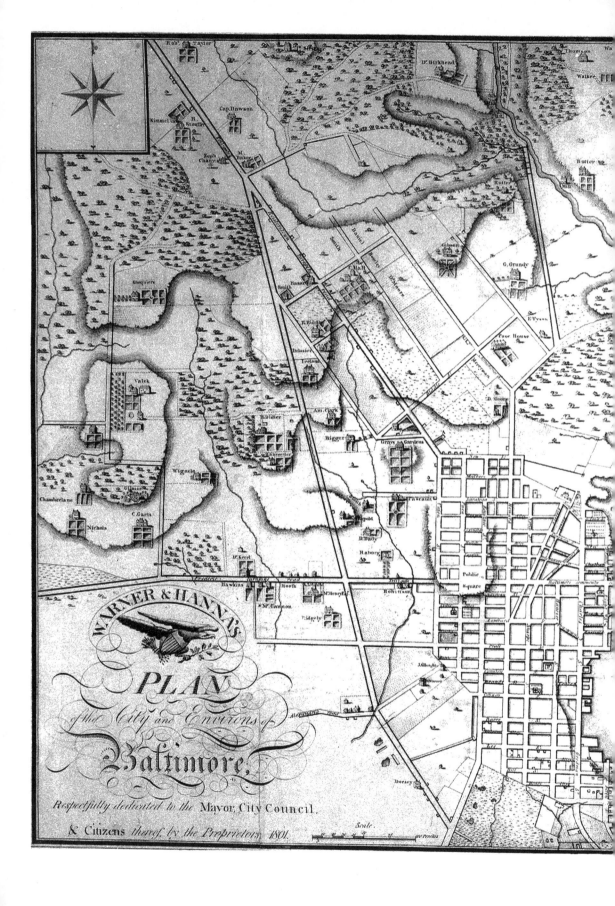

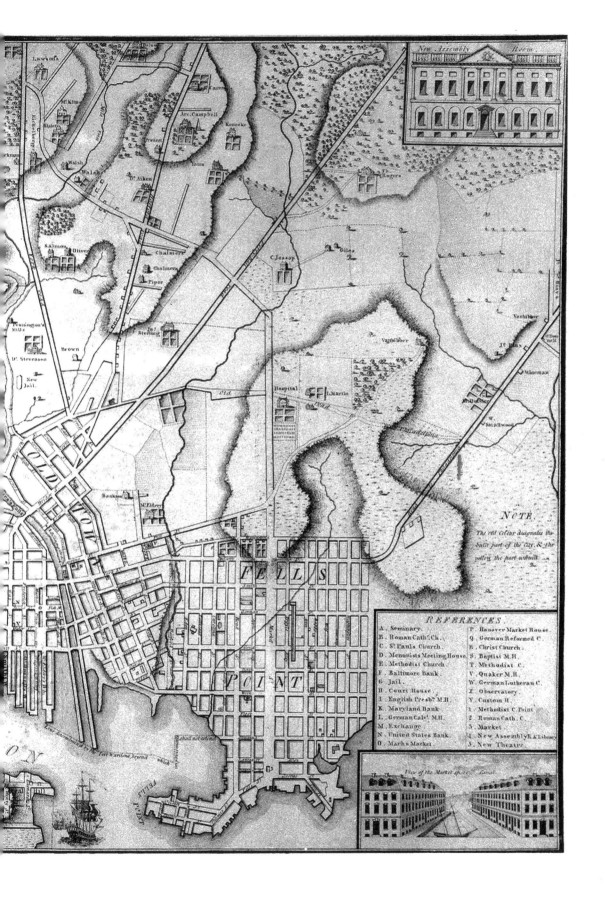

New Assembly Room.

REFERENCES.

A. Seminary.
B. Roman Cath. Ch.
C. St. Pauls Church.
D. Menonists Meeting House.
E. Methodist Church.
F. Baltimore Bank.
G. Jail.
H. Court House.
I. English Presb. M.H.
K. Maryland Bank.
L. German Calv. M.H.
M. Exchange.
N. United States Bank.
O. Marsh Market.

P. Hanover Market House.
Q. German Reformed C.
R. Christ Church.
S. Baptist M.H.
T. Methodist C.
V. Quaker M.H.
W. German Lutheran C.
X. Observatory.
Y. Custom H.
1. Methodist C. Point
2. Roman Cath. C.
3. Market.
4. New Assembly R. & Library.
5. New Theatre.

NOTE.
The red Colour designates the built part of the city, & the yellow the part unbuilt.

View of the Market space & Canal.

Charles Hodges of Thomas absent when drafted and called on a Jury.

The State of Maryland   Indictment for Murder.

vs

Negro Bob slave of   Non Cul and issue
Thomas Covington

Jury.   Witnesses sworn

1 Nicholas Young   Alexander Watson
2 John Hamilton Brown   John Hughes
3 Joseph Sansbury   William Wilson
4 Thomas Pownall   John Eastwood
5 Matthy Madson   Docter William Beanes
6 Hiram Belt   Trueman Tyler
7 James Belt
8 Thomas Clarkson
9 John Spalding   Verdict Guilty
10 William Hutcheson
11 John Burgess
12 John Thomas Wood

Ordered by the Court that Alexander Watson be allowed four Dollars for four days attendance at this Term as a Witness for the State against Negro Bob. —

Ordered by the Court that John Hughes be allowed three dollars for three days attendance at this Term as a Witness for the State of Maryland against Negro Bob. —

Ordered by the Court that William Wilson be allowed the sum of Three dollars for three days attendance at this Term as a Witness for the State against Negro Bob and three dollars for his Negro Man named Davy's attendance three days in same Case. —

Ordered that the Grand Jury be discharged. —

Benjamin Oden

vs   payment non payment and issue Def

George Newman   Verdict for Plantiff for   Witnesses sworn for Def.
                      £50.5 alof £15.165 6th Day Anthony Addison
Jury.   Judgment instr   William Sansbury
1 Thomas Baden   Appeal prayed to the Court acount of Jury.
2 John Thomas Wood   7 Basel Warton
3 Joseph Sansbury   8 John Spalding
4 John Burgess   9 Nicholas Young
5 John Evans   10 William Hutcheson
6 Thomas Young   11 Henry Brooke   } Talesmen
20 drawn and 8 strucken out.   12 Anthony Hardey

late 1807, the partially completed penitentiary was already being praised in a progress report as "that monument which the State has erected to its humanity and wisdom." Three acres had been purchased on the northeast edge of the city near the Jones Falls in what was then Baltimore County, where Madison and Forrest streets intersect today.[4] The commissioners had chosen the site carefully, "high and elevated, commanding an extensive and interesting prospect, and which must always enjoy a free circulation of air from its altitude over the surrounding grounds."[5] Fresh air was believed to be an important health measure that would help prevent yellow fever, which periodically ravaged the lowlands of nearby Fells Point. The "extensive and interesting prospect"—for whatever benefit it might have yielded to the convicts behind the twenty-foot-high walls—was soon to disappear as the penitentiary site was engulfed by the rapidly growing city.[6]

The exterior of the two buildings nearing completion was glowingly described in the same progress report as uniting "strength, simplicity and grandeur." The main building, for accommodating the guards and housing the warden and his family, was sixty feet square and three stories high. It was connected by a passage westward to a narrow dormitory wing (thirty-six feet wide and 156 feet long) for "the confinement of these unfortunate beings, whose crimes require that they should be excluded from the intercourse of society, . . . constructed to unite as much comfort and convenience as may be compatible with safety [i.e., security] and punishment." Each of the three floors had nine large night rooms (eight by fifteen feet, each holding seven to ten inmates) ranged along a hall extending the length of the building to admit light and air. Female convicts were housed in congregate cells separately from the men.[7] A chapel was provided—"in short, economy, utility and humanity appear to have been consulted in the erection and arrangement of the building." Clearly, the language of this progress report in 1807 reflects civic pride and self-satisfaction with what was then regarded as the most efficient and humane way of housing criminals.

Thomas McElderry and John Eager Howard and architects Robert Carey Long and Daniel Conn. The population of Baltimore doubled in the first decade of the nineteenth century. See Sherry Olson, *Baltimore: the Building of an American City* (Baltimore: Johns Hopkins University Press, 1980), p. 44.

[4] *Report of the Maryland Penitentiary Penal Commission* (Baltimore: State of Maryland, 1913), p. 307. Hereafter *Penal Commission Report*. J. Thomas Scharf, *History of Baltimore City and County* (Baltimore, 1881), p. 203.

[5] *Penal Commission Report*, p. 308.

[6] Olson, *Baltimore*, pp. 35, 54–56. See also the Poppleton map (1823) facing p. 64.

[7] The dimensions in this description come from Orlando Lewis, *The Development of American Prisons and Prison Customs, 1776–1845* [1922] (repr. Montclair, N.J.: Patterson Smith, 1967), p. 205.

Left: Prince George's County court docket from 1803, "State of Maryland vs. Negro Bob." (Maryland State Archives.)

Overleaf: First page of the prisoner reception book, misdated 1812 (the penitentiary opened in 1811). Note that most of the slaves had no surnames. Attempts at identification are imprecise. (Maryland State Archives 1878-0026.)

Names	Places of Nativity	Age	Complexion	Slave or not	Hair	Stature	Where placed
Negro Bob	Calvert County	22 years	Black	Slave	Black	5 - 6	Prince G.
Negro Will	Montgomery Co.	50 years	Yellow	Slave	Black	5 - 6	Montgom.
Negro Faraway	Anne Arundel Co.	23 years	Black	Slave	Black	5 - 8	A. Arundel
Joseph J. H. Caulk	Delaware	33 years	Dark		Dark	5 - 7	Talbot Co.
Negro Saml	Anne Arundel Co.	21 years	Black	Servant	Black	5 - 5	A. Arundel
Negro James	Montgomery Co.	31 years	Yellow	Slave	Black	5 - 4	Montgom.
Negro Joe	Harford County	24 years	Black	Slave	Black	5 - 8½	Baltimore
Negro Ham	Harford County	20 years	Black	Slave	Black	5 - 7	Baltimore
Negro Cyrus	Harford County	25 years	Black	Slave	Black	5 - 3	Baltimore
William Smith	Jamaica	Unknown	Black		Black	5 - 6	Baltimore
James Perry	Baltimore City	23 years	Fair		Brown	5 - 7½	Baltimore
James Linton	Sweden	20 years	Dark		Brown	5 - 4½	Washington
Negro James	St. Marys County	21 years	Black		Black	5 - 7	Cecil Co.
Negro Thomas alias James	Virginia	35 years	Black		Black	5 - 0½	District Co.
Negro Tom	Cecil County	27 years	Black	Slave	Black	6 - 1	Cecil Co.
Daniel Coker	Caroline County	26 years	Yellow		Grey	6 - 1½	Talbot Co.
Joseph Woodward	St. Marys County	30 years	Light		Brown	5 - 6½	Charles Co.
Major Truss	Worcester County	50 years	Black	Slave	Black	5 - 2	Baltimore
Nick Rice	Harford County	29 years	Black	Slave	Brown	5 - 7	Baltimore
Negro Harry	Anne Arundel Co.	21 years	Black	Slave	Black	5 - 8½	Baltimore
Jacob Lockler	Frederick County	29 years	Yellow	Slave	Black	5 - 6½	Frederick
Nicholas Queen	St. Marys County	37 years	Black		Black	5 - 7½	Frederick
Negro George	Frederick County	48 years	Black	Slave	Black	5 - 5	Frederick
Jonathan West	Frederick Co.	29 years	Dark		Brown	5 - 10½	Frederick
James Cunningham	Pennsylvania	24 years	Fair		Brown	5 - 6	Prince G.
Francis Piles	Prince Geo. County	29 years	Dark		Dark	5 - 9½	Prince G.
James Pryor	Queen Anns Co.	38 years	Black		Black	6 - 0	Queens Co.
Lew Tender	Talbot County	57 years	Black		Black	5 - 8	Talbot Co.
Negro James	Talbot County	18 years	Yellow	Slave	Black	5 - 6	Talbot Co.
Jon Cook	Frederick City	32 years	Dark		Sandy	5 - 5	Virginia
James Peloh	Harford City	36 years	Black	Slave	Black	5 - 6	Baltimore
Timothy Lynch	Ireland	40 years	Fair		Brown	5 - 6½	Baltimore
James Howell	Baltimore City	21 years	Yellow		Black	5 - 6	Baltimore
___ Kincaid	Ireland	38 years	Fair		Brown	5 - 7	State Pris...

Occupation	Marks	Counties where convicted	Crime	Date of Sentence
Labourer	Several Marks on the breast	Prince Geo. County	Murder	20 Octr. 1803
Labourer	None Perceivable	Anne Arundel Cty	Burglary & Larceny	16 April 1804
Sawyer	Scar on the right arm thick lip	Ditto	Burglary	16 Septr. 1805
Farmer	Wants right eye tooth	Talbot County	Murder	10 July 1809
Labourer	A small scar on the breast	Anne Arundel Cty	Assault with intent to commit a rape	13 Septr. 1809
Labourer	a scar in the upper lip	Montgomery Cty	Burglary &c	18 Novr. 1809
Labourer	Left little finger crooked	Harford County	Burglary	23 Decr. 1809
Labourer	Well made. No marks	Harford County	Burglary	23 Decr. 1809
Labourer	A scar near the left eye	Harford County	Burglary	23 Decr. 1809
Tailor	a mark on the neck. bent knee	Baltimore County	Larceny	17 Jany. 1810
Cooper	a scar each side the right knee	Baltimore County	Larceny	20 Jany. 1810
Sailor	PR marked on the left arm	Washington Cty	Horse Stealing	2 April 1810
Waiter	A scar on the left eye	Cecil County	Felony &c	4 April 1810
Sailor	A scar on the left jaw	Anne Arundel Cty	Larceny	16 April 1810
Labourer	Lusty finger. No marks	Cecil County	Manslaughter	11 Septr. 1810
Labourer	Left little finger crooked	Talbot County	Recg. Stolen Goods	12 Nov. 1810
Farmer	Slender made. no marks	Charles County	Horse Stealing	5 Septr. 1810
Wright	Scar of a burn on breast	Baltimore Cty	Burglary	22 Jany. 1811
Wright	Small scar right side the nose	Baltimore Cty	Burglary	22 Jany. 1811
Labourer	Short neck & round shoulders	Baltimore Cty	Assault with intent to murder	29 Jany. 1811
Labourer	A scar right side the nose	Frederick Cty	Larceny	22 Feby. 1811
Labourer	round shoulders, no marks	Frederick Cty	Larceny	22 Feby. 1811
Labourer	Wants several fore teeth	Frederick Cty	Larceny	22 Feby. 1811
Farmer	a scar left side the head	Frederick Cty	Larceny	22 Feby. 1811
Miller	The left ancle swelled	Prince Geo. Cty	Negro Stealing	13 April 1811
Farmer	Lusty. No marks	Prince Geo. Cty	Assault with intent to Murder	13 April 1811
Sailor	Remarkable scar on the left arm &c	Queen Anns Cty	Larceny	6 May 1811
Labourer	Scar on right hand &c	Talbot County	Larceny	1 June 1811
Labourer	Small spot on the left cheek	Talbot County	Felony	12 June 1811
Farmer	Wants the left eye	Baltimore Cty	Larceny	16 July 1811
Wright	right ancle smashed	Baltimore Cty	Burglary	19 July 1811
Labourer	a small mark. no marks	Baltimore Cty	Larceny	20 July 1811
Labourer	Smooth faced wild &c	Baltimore Cty	Larceny	29 July 1811
Tailor	Slender made. no marks	Baltimore Cty	Larceny	30 July 1811

The state's good intentions were also apparent when it came to the treatment of criminals. In setting down the rules for the government of the penitentiary in 1809, Maryland's General Assembly closely followed the rules—sometimes using the exact words (quoted below)—drawn up by the Philadelphia reformers for this country's first penitentiary department inside the Walnut Street Jail.[8] To prevent the spread of disease, convicts on admission were to be "separately washed and cleaned" and quarantined, their clothes to be "buried, baked, fumigated or carefully laid by," to be returned to them upon discharge. As for personal hygiene, prisoners were to wash their faces and hands every morning and before meals, change their linen at least once a week, be shaved once a week, and have their hair cut once a month. As for sanitation, the prison was to be "white-washed . . . at least twice in every year," swept out regularly and the prison yard "kept free from cows, hogs, dogs, and fowl." The rule of silence was laid down to prevent "evil communication": prisoners were forbidden to speak unless first spoken to and then only to authorized persons. Males and females were to be kept apart at all times. Prisoners were expected to earn their keep through productive labor. The employment of each prisoner was to be "such as the keeper may consider the best adapted to his or her age, sex, and state of health, having due regard to the employment which is most profitable." Both institutions used the carrot-and-stick approach to maintaining discipline. Prisoners who distinguished themselves "by their attention to cleanliness, sobriety, industry, and orderly conduct" would be "reported to the inspectors, and meet with such reward" as was "in their power to grant or procure for them." Any prisoners "found remiss or negligent in performing the work required" or who wasted or damaged materials would be punished by solitary confinement and reduced food allowance. And both institutions made provision for the care of the bodies and souls of prisoners. A physician was assigned to look after their health, and all prisoners were required to attend divine worship on Sunday except those who were sick. How strictly these rules were enforced is difficult to determine from this distance in time, but as is shown by how closely Baltimore followed Philadelphia's phrasing, the Maryland legislature took some pains to imitate the best example of prison management then known.[9]

That is not to say the imitation was slavish. The rules set down by the Maryland lawmakers were more numerous and more elaborate than those of the early

---

[8]*The Acts of Assembly . . . and the Rules and Regulations Respecting the Penitentiary of Maryland* (Baltimore, 1819), p. 24, and Negley K. Teeters, *The Cradle of the Penitentiary* (Philadelphia, 1955), p. 133, appendix 4.

[9]In the following citation, roman numerals refer to regulations in *The Acts of Assembly . . . and the Rules and Regulations Respecting the Penitentiary of Maryland* (Baltimore, 1819), p. 24, and arabic numbers refer to "The First Body of Rules Drawn Up for the Walnut Street Prison February 26, 1792," Appendix 4, p. 133, in Teeters, *Cradle of the Penitentiary:* XXIV-9, IV-13, XXV-14, X-15 and 16, VI-1, II-2, XIII-3 and 4, VIII-12, XL-7, XXXVI-17, and XIX-18.

AN INQUIRY,

WHETHER

CRIME AND MISERY

ARE

PRODUCED OR PREVENTED, BY OUR PRESENT SYSTEM

OF

Prison Discipline.

ILLUSTRATED BY DESCRIPTIONS OF

THE BOROUGH COMPTER.	THE JAILS AT BURY & ILCHESTER.
TOTHILL FIELDS PRISON.	THE MAISON DE FORCE AT GHENT.
THE JAIL AT ST. ALBANS.	THE PHILADELPHIA PRISON.
THE JAIL AT GUILDFORD.	THE PENITENTIARY AT MILLBANK.
THE JAIL AT BRISTOL.	AND THE PROCEEDINGS OF THE
	LADIES' COMMITTEE AT NEWGATE.

By THOMAS FOWELL BUXTON.

" I make no scruple to affirm, that if it were the aim and wish of Magistrates to effect the destruction, present and future, of young delinquents, they could not desire a more effectual method than to confine them in our Prisons."—HOWARD.

" Whereas, if many offenders convicted of crimes, for which transportation has been usually inflicted, were ordered for solitary confinement, accompanied by well-regulated labour and religious instruction, it might be the means, under Providence, not only of deterring others from the commission of the like Crimes, but also of reforming the individuals, and inuring them to habits of Industry, &c."—19 GEORGE III. c. 74. s. 8.

SECOND EDITION.

London:

PRINTED FOR JOHN AND ARTHUR ARCH, CORNHILL; BUTTERWORTH AND SONS, FLEET STREET; AND JOHN HATCHARD, PICCADILLY.

1818.

As the penitentiary sought to establish its rules and discipline, British reformer Thomas Fowell Buxton, who had investigated the Pennsylvania penitentiary in Philadelphia, published his *Inquiry*. (Maryland Historical Society.)

Abstract of Prisoners received into the Maryland Penitentiary from the 1st of December, 1817, to the 30th of November, 1818, inclusive.

CRIMES.

- 92 Stealing,
- 4 House breaking,
- 3 Passing co'trf'it b'nk notes,
- Felony,
- 14 Vagrancy,
- 1 Horse stealing,
- 1 Perjury,
- 4 Receiving stolen goods,
- 2 Attempt to ravish,
- 1 Exciting insurrection,
- 1 Manslaughter,
- 5 Kidnapping,
- 1 Rape,
- 2 Murder 2d degree,
- 2 Arson,
- 1 Assault with intent to kill,
- 146

Column headings of the abstract: Whites (Men, Women); Blacks (Men, Women); Americans — Maryland, New-York, New Jersey, Pennsylvania, Massachusetts, Delaware, Connecticut, Dist. Columbia, Virginia, Vermont, Wales; Foreigners — Ireland, Island Guarnzy, England, France, Holland, Africa, Scotland; Counties where convicted — Baltimore, Washington, Montgomery, Charles, Harford, Caroline, Frederick, St. M'y's, Dorchester, Prince George, Anne-Arundel, Somerset, Queen-Anne's, Worcester, Cecil, Talbot.

Of 146 Prisoners received,

8 were for 3 months
1 was for 4
4 were for 6
1 was for 10
1 for 13
55 were for 1 year,
25 for 2
13 for 3
30 for 4
5 for 5
5 for 6
5 for 7
11 for 8
5 for 15
1 was for 18
146

Of 77 natives of Maryland,

3 were born in Frederick county
4 in Montgomery
4 in Charles
4 in Queen-Anne's
4 in Prince-George's
16 in Baltimore
8 in Harford
8 in Dorchester
5 in St. Mary's
5 in Anne-Arundel
5 in Calvert
5 in Kent
7 in Caroline
11 in Washington
5 in Somerset
2 in Worcester
2 in Cecil
1 in Talbot
77

Prisoners discharged from the 1st December, 1817, to the 30th November, 1818, inclusive.

95 their time of confinement having expired
17 by pardon
21 died
133

305 prisoners remained in the penitentiary on the 30th November, 1817,
146 were received from the 1st Dec. 1817, to the 30th Nov. 1818, inclusive.
451
133 were discharged as above
318 remaining in the penitentiary.

December 1st, 1818.

Inventory of the Goods on hand belonging to the Mary-land Penitentiary, November 30th, 1818.

Cordwaining Account.

133	Sheep skins	$199 50
12	Wax calf, do.	40 00
12	Morocco, do.	18 00
19	Sides coarse leather,	28 50
42	Do. Fine,	63 00
547lb.	Sole,	158 63
1	pair boot legs,	1 50
872	do. Shoes various kinds in store,	554 50
1	Lot of soal leather,	50 00
76	Sides do. unbroken,	385 70
157	Pair mens' uppers closed,	117 75
31	Dozen womens'. do	155 00
	Sundry other articles, implements and furniture,	603 94
		———— 2376 02

Smith and Nailing Account.

Sundry lots new and old iron, chains, implements and shop
furniture, amounting to   1209 11

Sawing Account.

Sundry saws, boxes sand, and other articles,   749 50

Hatting Account.

125	Napped hats, unfinished,	281 25
8	Roram, do. do.	24 00
30	Wool, do. do.	20 00
2	Castors, do. do.	14 00
83	Wool, do. do.	54 78
36	do. damaged,	15 00
60	Napped bodies uncoloured,	100 00
50	Napping, do. do.	25 00
100	Felt, do. do.	50 00
100	Muskrat skins,	33 33
241	Bound hats,	90 37
59	Roram hat bodies,	35 40
1050lbs.	Danish wool, at 50 cts.	525 00
648lbs.	Roram, do. do.	324 00
2850lbs.	Felt, do. 25 cts.	712 50
	Sundry other articles, such as lining, bands, leather, dye stuff, shop furniture, &c.	778 07
82	Fine and wool hats in store,	173 25
		———— 3255 97

Dyeing Account.

36lb.	Bengal indigo,	63 00
300	do. Green copperas,	9 00

Abstract of prisoners received in the first eleven months of 1818 (opposite), and a portion of the recorded inventory, from the *Annual Report of the Inspectors of the Penitentiary, 1817/1818* (above). Copy at the Enoch Pratt Free Library, Baltimore. The penitentiary's goal to be self-supporting meant that whenever possible careful inventory records were kept.

reformers in Philadelphia. For example, convicts were to be "clothed in habits of coarse materials, uniform in colour and make, and distinguishing them from the good citizens of this state." They were to be "sustained upon bread, Indian meal, or other inferior food . . . and allowed two meals of coarse meat in each week." Working hours for the prisoners were spelled out in detail: they were to labor every day except Sunday and Christmas Day, the daily hours being eight in November, December, and January, nine in February and October, and ten during the other months. Habits of industry ("an evidence of reformation") were to be encouraged by individual accounts being kept for prisoners. Misbehavior could be punished by the "keeper" (warden) with solitary confinement on bread and water for a period "not exceeding ten days"; for more serious offenses, the board of "inspectors" (directors) could order "moderate whipping or . . . repeated whipping, not exceeding thirteen lashes."[10]

Such treatment of prisoners today would evoke howls of protest from inside the walls and outside as well. But at the time it was intended as an improvement over the treatment of prisoners in workhouses, jails, and prisons both here and abroad before the reforms of the late eighteenth century.[11] Among other things, prisoners entering the new Maryland Penitentiary would be clothed, fed, and given medical care at public expense and pay no fees or "garnish" to their keepers. And though they were expected to pay for their maintenance through productive labor, they would have the chance to earn some money for themselves through "overtask" (exceeding their daily quotas), which would be given to them upon discharge to help them get started in a better life.[12]

Punishment was no longer left to the whim of the keepers but prescribed according to the nature of the offense. Solitary confinement for misbehavior was regarded as more humane than the varieties of corporal punishment (stocks, pillory, branding, etc.) inflicted in the past.[13] And though whipping was still used for serious offenses, it was supposed to be "moderate and carefully regulated" (ordered by the board of "inspectors") and "not extending to life or limb."[14]

Aside from being one of the punishments, confinement in a solitary cell for at least a part of one's sentence was also an essential feature of the new penitentiary

---

[10] *Acts of Assembly . . .* (1819), Regulations XXIX, XXX and XXXI, and XL.

[11] For an extended description of the treatment of prisoners before the reforms, see Robin Evans, *The Fabrication of Virtue: English Prison Architecture, 1750–1840* (Cambridge: Cambridge University Press, 1982), chapters one and two.

[12] *Acts of Assembly . . .* (1819), Regulation XXI.

[13] Michel Foucault, *Discipline and Punish: The Birth of the Prison* (New York: Pantheon, 1977), pp. 10, 124.

[14] *Acts of Assembly . . .* (1819), Regulations XXXII and XL. Whipping gradually fell into disuse as the nineteenth century wore on but persisted in some states, notably Delaware, until well into the twentieth century. See Robert Caldwell, *Red Hannah: Delaware's Whipping Post* (Philadelphia: University of Pennsylvania Press, 1947), p. 1.

idea: to allow the prisoner to reflect on his past misdeeds. Once removed from the possibly corrupting influence of other prisoners, he was expected to see the error of his ways and reform himself accordingly.[15] But single cells were much more costly to build than congregate cells, and therefore relatively few single cells were to be found in the construction of the first penitentiaries. The Maryland Penitentiary's first dormitory wing, which could house 360 prisoners, was constructed with only nine single cells.[16] Solitary confinement was used there in the early years mainly for punishing unruly prisoners.[17]

Along with solitary confinement, hard labor had been incorporated into the new penitentiary idea because of the corrective morality believed to be inherent in work.[18] After "Negro Bob" Butler and his fellow convicts had gone through the reception process of being bathed, deloused, and issued coarse brown garb and had been settled in their congregate cells, they were given work supposedly suited to their individual skills and capacities. In view of his age (twenty-two) and height (five feet, six inches) and former occupation as a laborer,[19] young Butler was probably put to work sawing marble in the stone shed rather than performing tasks requiring more skill, such as weaving, cordwaining (boot-and-shoe making), or comb-and-brushmaking. As female convicts entered the new penitentiary, they were housed in separate wards of the dormitory wing (six rooms at the southern end of the second story[20]) and labored in a separate yard at spinning, knitting, and laundry, and forbidden all communication with male convicts. Racial segregation, however, does not appear to have been practiced at the penitentiary during the very early years.[21] Prisoners of both sexes labored from sunrise to sunset with a half hour off for breakfast and one hour for dinner. Supper was served immediately following the closing of the shops, and at nine o'clock the lamps were extinguished and the convicts were locked in their cells for the night.[22]

The penitentiary was governed by the keeper and a board of twelve inspectors (later called directors), all of whom were appointed by the governor of the state and his council. Apart from being responsible for prison discipline, the keeper—acting with the approval of the board of directors—was to contract for the clothing and diet of the convicts as well as for the materials and tools used by them to

---

[15]Foucault, *Discipline and Punish,* pp. 122–23, and Evans, *Fabrication of Virtue,* pp. 73–74, 119.

[16]Lewis, *Development of American Prisons,* p. 205.

[17]A letter from the penitentiary board of directors said that solitary confinement had been used only for punishment from the very beginning. See *Journal of the House of Delegates* (1822), p. 141.

[18]Foucault, *Discipline and Punish,* pp. 121–22, and Evans, *Fabrication of Virtue,* p. 119.

[19]Maryland Penitentiary, Reception Records, #5655, Maryland Hall of Records.

[20]Lewis, *Development of American Prisons,* p. 205.

[21]Marvin Gettleman, "The Maryland Penitentiary in the Age of Tocqueville, 1828–1842," *Maryland Historical Magazine,* 56 (1961): 276.

[22]*Acts of the Assembly . . .* (1819), Regulations XXX and XLVIII.

manufacture goods, which were sold in the open market. From the sale of such goods the keeper was to receive a 5 percent commission which went toward making up part of his annual salary of $1,000. Each of his assistant keepers (appointed by him and numbering up to eight) received $250 annually. A bookkeeper, appointed by the board of directors, took charge of the penitentiary records for an annual salary of $500.[23]

In order to discourage corrupt management or the abuse of prisoners, an elaborate system of supervision and accountability was put in place. Two of the directors were to visit the penitentiary every week to examine its management, supplemented by an inspection visit from six court-appointed grand jurors during every law term. The keeper of the penitentiary was required to submit quarterly and annual reports to the board of directors, who in turn were to report annually to the governor, who then reported to the General Assembly.[24]

Careful records appear to have been kept at the penitentiary from the very beginning, some of which have survived to the present day. The manuscript pages of the first reception books, for example, were divided into neatly ruled columns for data regarding the prisoner: name, place of residence, occupation, identifying marks, county where convicted, crime, and date of sentence. Though the descriptions of distinguishing features usually lacked precision by today's standards (Bob Butler had "several natural marks on the breast"), at least some effort was made and certain notations have a quaint ring to them (Joseph Caulk: "Wants right eye tooth" or Daniel Coker: "Left little finger crooked").[25]

Among the early published records that have survived are some revealing statistics relating to the makeup of the prison population and crime and punishment for the years 1812 through 1832 appended to English visitor William Crawford's *Report on the Penitentiaries of the U.S.* (1835).[26] During the penitentiary's first full year of operation (1812), ninety-two additional prisoners were committed, some of them mere boys and therefore at the mercy of older, hardened convicts (at the time no reformatories for juvenile offenders existed):

Under 16 years old	–	6
16 to 20	–	11
20 to 30	–	33
30 to 40	–	25
40 & upwards	–	17

---

[23]Ibid., Regulations XXXVIII, XLII, and p. 37.
[24]Ibid., pp. 28, 31, 47–48.
[25]Maryland Penitentiary, Reception Records #5655, p. 1, Maryland State Archives.
[26](Reprinted Montclair, N.J.: Patterson-Smith, 1969), pp. 98–101.

Eleven of these new prisoners were slaves, whose market value had been determined by the court where they had been convicted and then paid to their owners.[27] From 1812 through 1832 there were twenty-four hangings. Five crimes were listed as punishable by death: murder, rape, arson, treason, and insurrection by free blacks or slaves. As might be expected, such lesser offenses as burglary, larceny, assault, and forgery were punishable by prison terms of varying length, but some of the offenses would hardly seem to justify such punishment today: vagrancy, gambling, and bestiality. Certain offenses vividly evoke the turbulent life of the times: horse-stealing, dueling, enticing slaves to run away, tarring and feathering, and cutting or stealing any buoy in the Chesapeake Bay or Patapsco River (done by land pirates in order to shipwreck a vessel and then plunder it).

Few of the very early published annual reports of the penitentiary's board of directors and the warden to the governor—containing financial statistics—have survived, apparently only four of those published before 1828.[28] Nevertheless, enough information can be garnered from other published sources to show the importance of prison labor to the financial health of the fledgling institution. Miscellaneous workshops and sheds were built throughout the prison for such industries as weaving (on hand looms) and dyeing woolen and cotton goods, cordwaining (boot and shoemaking), hatting, nailmaking, comb and brushmaking, and sawing marble and limestone—diverse enough so that all prisoners could be employed except the most infirm.[29]

Despite this determined effort to keep as many prisoners working as possible, the penitentiary failed during its first decade to meet one of its two main goals: to support itself financially through the productive labor of its inmates. By November 30, 1819, it had already run up a debt of $39,126.25, not because of mismanagement by the board of directors, a legislative committee reported, but as the result of such varied causes as organizational problems natural to a new institution with regard to prison labor, lack of experience in policing the penitentiary, and depressed trade conditions. Its shaky financial condition was not helped by a fire, believed to be arson, that seriously damaged the dormitory wing on March 5, 1817.[30] Yet the committee hoped that improved management of prison labor would soon make the institution self-supporting.[31] Indeed, it soon became so. A

---

[27]An act passed by the Assembly in 1818 may have eliminated slaves (but not free blacks) from the prison population. Instead, the offender was to be hanged, flogged, or banished from the state. See Gettleman, "Maryland Penitentiary in the Age of Tocqueville," p. 276, n26.

[28]Enoch Pratt Free Library has the *Annual Report* for 1817/18. The Maryland Historical Society Library has reports for 1822, 1823, and 1825.

[29]These industries are listed in the earliest surviving annual report for 1817/18, pp. 5–7. Numerous other industries would be added in future years. See the long list in the *Penal Commission Report* (1913), p. 310.

[30]*Niles' Weekly Register,* March 8, 1817, p. 32, reported an estimated loss of $12,000–15,000.

[31]*Journal of the House of Delegates* (1820), p. 35.

(8)

Q. Do you consider the keeper qualified to perform the duties of his office?

A. I do not think him in any manner fit for the situation.

Q. Will you state your general reasons for thinking him incompetent?

A. He wants talents, industry and energy.

RACHAEL PERRIGO, was sworn.

Q. Have you any knowledge of the duties of the keeper?

A. I have.

Q. How are they performed?

A. They are not performed in the manner required by law?

Q. Is the keeper vigilant and industrious in the discharge of his duties?

A. He is not.

Q. Have any differences existed between you and the keeper?

A. There have.

Q. Have the persons under your charge the advantage of religious instruction.

A. They have on every Sabbath morning at my request.

(9)

Dr. WM. W. WALLS, was sworn.

Q. Does the keeper of the Penitentiary afford you all the facilities necessary to a satisfactory discharge of your professional duties in the institution.

A. He does not. Instead of assisting he rather embarasses my operations.

Q. In your visits to the house have you been able to discover any improper conduct of the keeper or other officers?

A. I have not.

Q. Do you think that the keeper is a man of capacity, industry, truth and honor, and such as the keeper of the Penitentiary should be?

A. I do not think him entitled to that character.

Q. What is your opinion of the book-keeper and agent; and what of the matron of the female department, with the prisoners under whose charge you must of course have had professional intercourse?

A. The book-keeper and agent are men of capacity, and fitted for the situations they hold. The matron is also qualified for her situation.

2

Early dissension in the penitentiary administration, 1823. In 1822 the penitentiary hired a matron, the first in the United States, to supervise female inmates. Mrs. Rachael Perijo (or Perrigo) quickly brought order and financial self-sufficiency to her department, but fell afoul of Warden Nathaniel Hynson, who described her as competent but "highly tempered." In the pages above, prison physician William W. Walls joined her in testifying before a legislative committee about their differences with Warden Hynson, whose staff described him almost unanimously as honest but lazy, and a poor disciplinarian. His tenure lasted until 1825. (From *Depositions Taken at the Penitentiary by the Committee Appointed for that Purpose by the Legislature of Maryland* [Annapolis: J. Hughes, Printer, ca. 1823]. Maryland Historical Society.)

period of "very remarkable prosperity" lay ahead, from 1822 to 1839, during which time prison industries enabled the penitentiary to be not only self-supporting but a highly profitable institution that could finance much of its growth internally.[32]

The penitentiary during its first decade also failed to meet expectations regarding its other main purpose: reformation of its convicts. In the female department, occupying six rooms of the second story at the southern end of the dormitory wing, sixty or so convicts slept ten to a room, two or three to a bed, which gave rise to "some vile abuses practised among them." More significantly, as in other prisons, the department had been managed by a male keeper—"wretchedly" so, as the directors themselves admitted. However, in February 1822, Mrs. Rachael Perijo (Perrigo, elsewhere) was placed in charge, the first prison matron in this country of whom there is any record. Her management over the next three years was hailed as exemplary in the annual *Report of the Prison Discipline Society of Boston* (1826).[33] She turned the department's average annual deficit of $1,099 into an average surplus of $492, improved the discipline, health, and morale of her charges, taught them useful trades and, with the help of her daughter, how to read, and encouraged them in religious worship. Her enlightened and energetic supervision was said to have resulted in an "unusually small" number of recommitments. But it also apparently gave rise to a feud between her and the keeper, Nathaniel Hynson, who was almost unanimously described by his staff as a poor disciplinarian, honest but lazy.[34]

The reformation or discipline of the majority of the prison population—approximately 250 male convicts—remained a stubborn problem mainly because of their greater numbers and the corrupting effect of "evil communication." During the day these convicts labored together in workshops that were scattered throughout the institution and therefore difficult to keep under close surveillance. At night they were crowded eight or ten to a room, the youthful along with the hardened offenders, and left to their own devices. "Much insubordination, and occasional disorders were the natural and unavoidable consequences," the directors said, "which no skill or conduct of the keeper and his deputies could possibly prevent."[35] The few incidents reported in Baltimore's only news magazine were undoubtedly only the tip of the iceberg. On the morning of August 28, 1820,

---

[32] *Report of the Committee on Prison Manufacturing of the Maryland Penitentiary* (Baltimore, 1842), p. 4.

[33] (Reprinted Montclair, N.J.: Patterson Smith, 1972), pp. 34–35, and Lewis, *Development of American Prisons,* p. 205.

[34] *Depositions Taken at the Penitentiary by the Committee Appointed for that purpose by the Legislature of Maryland* [ca. 1823], p. 4. On his side, Hynson testified that Mrs. Perijo was competent "but a highly tempered woman."

[35] *Testimony Taken Before the Joint Committee of the Legislature on the Penitentiary* (Baltimore, 1837), p. 9.

> *Maryland penitentiary.* An extensive system for forging or altering the denominations of bank notes, was recently discovered within the walls of this institution!—a deputy keeper was in the plot, and the agent who carried on the business. Thirteen plates, or rather parts of plates, were found; but it is supposed that a good many of their manufactures were put in circulation, purporting to be of the Frederick County bank.

This account of a counterfeiting ring operating within the new penitentiary astounded the editors of *Niles' Weekly Register* and presumably the holders of notes issued by the Frederick County bank. (*Niles Weekly Register,* September 7, 1822, Maryland Historical Society.)

according *Niles' Weekly Register* (September 2), a "desperate" escape attempt took place, during which one convict was killed and several more severely wounded by the keepers. And on September 7, 1822, the magazine reported the discovery of a large forgery operation involving one of the deputy keepers. A report of a legislative committee called the penitentiary at this time "a nursery of crime," principally because single-cell confinement, which it considered the only valuable feature of the penitentiary system, was seldom carried out. A vicious criminal, it went on to say, should not be allowed to associate with others like himself "to plot and execute new crimes, as has been the case in the Maryland Penitentiary, but closely confined with only as much light as will enable him to read the bible which should be his sole companion; then there will be a chance for reformation."[36]

Because single cells were more expensive to build than congregate cells, only twenty-two existed at the Maryland Penitentiary, not nearly enough to carry out one of the original aims of the penitentiary system: confinement of each convict for a time in a single cell so that he could reflect on his criminal past, see the error of his ways, and reform himself accordingly. In common with other penitentiaries before 1820, the Maryland institution had used its relatively few single cells only to isolate its more unruly convicts. To provide enough single cells for all convicts—thereby preventing "evil association"—an additional building would be needed. On March 6, 1827, a select legislative committee reported that it had drafted a bill authorizing the directors of the penitentiary to erect another building and the Maryland treasurer to raise the money for it by loan.[37]

[36] *Journal of the House of Delegates* (1822), pp. 139–40.
[37] *Journal of the House of Delegates* (1826), p. 458. When the penitentiary opened in 1811, its dormitory had

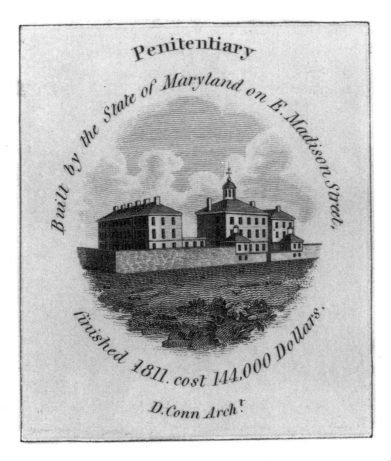

The penitentiary as depicted in a margin vignette on a post-1829 edition of Thomas Poppleton's map of Baltimore. (Maryland Historical Society.)

The design of the Maryland Penitentiary's new building was determined by
the choice made by the state between two competing systems of single-cell confinement aimed at eliminating "evil association." The first had evolved at the state
prison at Auburn, New York, and the other at the Eastern State Penitentiary at
Philadelphia. Basically, the two systems differed as follows: at Auburn, the prisoners were isolated in small (seven feet by three and one-half feet) individual cells
only during the night and worked during the day in congregate shops and ate
together under close surveillance and a strictly enforced (by the lash) rule of silence. At Philadelphia, the prisoners were completely isolated both night and day
in individual cells large enough (eleven feet, nine inches long by seven feet, six
inches wide) for them to eat, sleep, and work.[38]

---

only nine single cells (Lewis, *Development of American Prisons*, p. 205). Thirteen more cells appear to have been
subsequently created by converting two of the congregate night rooms.

[38]Lewis, *Development of American Prisons*, p. 124.

While the Philadelphia system did prevent the promiscuous intermingling of prisoners, it was expensive, each cell costing $1,200 compared to $150 in the Auburn system, a ratio of eight to one.[39] Moreover, the handcraft prison labor carried on in the cells of the Philadelphia system was inefficient and less productive than the congregate workshops equipped with power machinery of the Auburn system.[40] Mainly for economic reasons, Maryland, along with most other penitentiaries in the United States,[41] adopted the Auburn system of isolating convicts at night and the rule of silence while they worked together during the day.

The new east dormitory wing, costing $36,086, was designed by William F. Small, with some help from the Reverend Louis Dwight, president of the Boston Prison Discipline Society. It was built largely by convict labor[42] of brick, measured 40 feet by 170 feet, and had five stories (including its half-sunk basement story). Its 320 cells were ranged along the outside walls (the so-called "outside construction," used at Philadelphia) and faced each other across a hall fifteen feet wide. This arrangement, which allowed for windows, gave the cells more light and air than the cellblocks at Auburn, in which windowless cells were placed inside back-to-back down the center ("inside construction"). Additional benefits were supposed to accrue from the new dormitory's arcade interior, constructed according to a plan by the Reverend Mr. Dwight. Instead of floors for the upper stories, three-feet-wide galleries ran in front of each range of cells, leaving the center of the hall open to its arched roof. The design, the *Annual Report* of 1828 confidently asserted, "will enable the guard in the lower story, to observe, at the same time, the door of every cell: by this means, rendering the escape of any convict impossible." The interior was heated by three large stoves equidistant on the floor of the hall, and light was provided by nine lanterns.[43]

Each cell measured eight feet, six inches long; three feet, seven inches wide; and seven feet high. Light and air were admitted through a glazed window in the outer wall, measuring three feet high and four inches wide on the wall's outer face (to prevent escape), broadening to twelve inches on the inner surface. Each cell

---

[39] *North American Review* (July 1839): 39.

[40] Harry Elmer Barnes and Negley K. Teeters, *New Horizons in Criminology,* 3rd ed. (Englewood Cliffs, N.J.: Prentice-Hall, Inc., 1959), p. 342.

[41] The Philadelphia system met with more approval in European countries. See Barnes and Teeters, *New Horizons,* pp. 344–46.

[42] Carpentry, smithing, painting and plastering. See *Annual Report* (1829). See also *Index to Laws of Maryland* (1827 session), chap. 37, sect. 3.

[43] *Annual Report* (1828), p. 10. The physical details for the new dormitory came from the board of directors' *Reports* of 1828 and 1829; William Crawford, *Report on the Penitentiaries of the U.S.* (1835), p. 94; M. Demetz and Abel Blouet, *Rapport à Monsieur le Comte de Montalivet sur les pénitenciers des États-Unis* (Paris: Imprimerie Royale, 1837), p. 36; Lewis, *Development of American Prisons,* p. 206; and the Boston Prison Discipline Society, *Fourth Annual Report* (1829), p. 265.

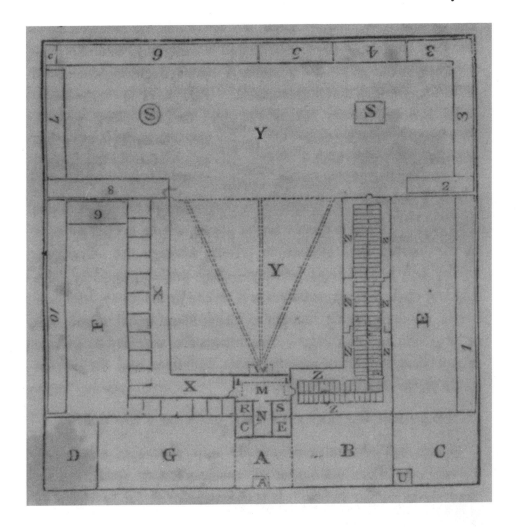

"Ground View of the Auburn [New York] Prison." When the Maryland Penitentiary decided to build a new dormitory, a committee went north to visit the penitentiaries and prisons in Philadelphia, the state prison at Sing Sing, and the new penitentiary at Auburn, New York. After studying the Auburn design, the committee concluded that "labour by day and solitary confinement at night, is the best sytem that has been devised for the punishment of criminals. . . . it is the most economical in practice, and the most effectual in producing reformation." The committee adopted the Auburn design with modifications. When the penitentiary built the east dormitory (later "G" dormitory), it constructed narrow cells like those seen at right center above but did not place them back-to-back. Instead, they created an arcade interior in which one guard in the center could view all the cells. (From *Report of the Committee Appointed by the Board of Directors of the Maryland Penitentiary, To Visit the Penitentiaries and Prisons in the City of Philadelphia and State of New York* [Baltimore: Lucas & Deaver, Printer, 1828].)

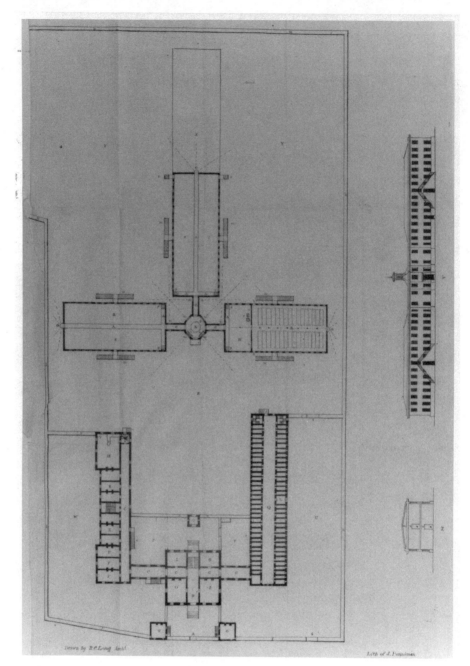

An architectural drawing made by Robert Cary Long shows the two stages in the early development of the penitentiary. First, the original square administration building (bottom) and west dormitory with its large congregate nightrooms (eight by fifteen feet, each holding seven to ten prisoners). Second, the later adoption of the Auburn system of single-cell confinement, whereby prisoners were isolated in small (seven by three and one-half feet) individual cells (east dormitory) only at night, working during the day in congregate workshops under close surveillance. Inspection corridors can be seen running down the centers of the north and west wings of the radial workshops from the octagonal keeper's office. The east wing contained a kitchen, dining room, and chapel. From *Report of the Committee of Directors, . . .* 1835.

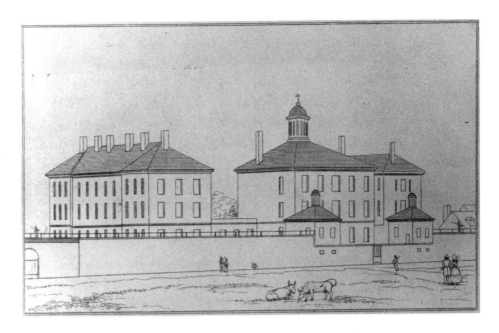

This sketch of the penitentiary, made in 1832, shows the square administration building (1811) flanked by its two dormitory wings, western (1811) and eastern (1829), in open fields near the Jones Falls. The rapidly growing city soon engulfed this pastoral setting. (Maryland Historical Society.)

had an iron slatted door with a slat extending to a staple beyond the reach of the prisoner where it was fastened by a padlock in common with the slat of the neighboring cell. Furnishings were Spartan: a cot with sacking bottom, a mattress filled with waste yarn, three blankets, a coverlet of cotton and wool, a can of water, a covered "filth" bucket, and—a bible.[44] Six "dark" cells, equipped with venetian shutters, were set aside in the basement story for punishment. Offenders were flogged and then locked in both day and night on a reduced diet.[45]

With the completion of the east dormitory wing in 1829, the state had taken the first step in adopting the Auburn system. The separation of male convicts at night was expected to produce "a great improvement" in discipline.[46] But while the male prisoners were physically separated from sunset to sunrise, the slatted doors of their facing cells did not prevent communication. The British visitor William Crawford observed in 1833: "The prisoners can talk together from cell to cell and make signs to those opposite."[47]

During the day, when the male convicts worked and ate together, the Auburn rule of silence was supposed to be rigidly enforced. According to Crawford:

[44]Crawford, *Penitentiaries of the U.S.,* p. 95.
[45]Demetz and Blouet, *les pénitenciers des États Unis,* p. 36.
[46]*Annual Report of the Boston Prison Discipline Society* (1829), p. 264.
[47]*Penitentiaries of the U.S.,* p. 94, n3.

> The prisoners are marched to and from their cells and workshops with the close lock-step in silence, their heads being all turned one way. . . . At their meals the prisoners sit down and rise up at the ringing of a bell. The tables are arranged in such a manner as to prevent the men facing each other. . . . The officers watch the prisoners closely at their meals to prevent communication, and such as are detected in holding intercourse, are flogged.

But the English visitor found the discipline to be "extremely lax" compared to that at Auburn. The prisoners still managed to communicate during their brief visits to the pumps and privies in the yard and especially in the workshops, where they spent most of their time.[48] Adequate supervision of these workshops was "impracticable," according to the board of directors' annual report in 1834, because of their irregular construction, scattered location throughout the prison, and division into numerous rooms. Acting on the board's recommendation, the state now took the second step for the full implementation of the Auburn system: during the 1834/5 session, the General Assembly authorized the construction of a complex of workshops especially designed for more effective surveillance of the prisoners while at work during the day. Ground was broken in May 1835.[49]

Completed early in 1836 at a cost of $50,000,[50] the new workshops for male convicts were designed by Baltimore architect Robert Carey Long, who copied the radial plan used by John Haviland for the cellhouses at Philadelphia's Eastern Penitentiary.[51] Long laid out three rectangular two-story wings, to the north (measuring 150 by 50 feet), east, and west (the latter two measuring 106 by 50 feet), connected by corridors to a central octagonal pavilion, the keeper's office. From this office the keeper or his assistants could enter a box-like inspection corridor that ran down the center of the north and west wings (the east wing contained a kitchen, dining room, and chapel) and look into each workshop through a narrow, horizontal, six-inch slit. There, according to a pair of official visitors from France who toured the facility, prisoners and guards alike performed their duties "knowing that an invisible eye could discover their least movement." The latrines were located in a small tower at the end of each wing. A system was devised to

---

[48]Ibid., p. 95.

[49]*Testimony Taken Before the Joint Committee of the Legislature on the Penitentiary* (Baltimore, 1837), pp. 11–12.

[50]Ibid., p. 12.

[51]Robert Carey Long (1810–49), also designed the City Jail (erected 1832), St. Timothy's Episcopal Church in Catonsville (1845), and the Lloyd Street Synagogue (1845). See Henry F. Withey, *Biographical Dictionary of American Architects (Deceased)* (Los Angeles: New Age Publishing Co., 1956), p. 378, and Neal A. Brooks and Richard Parsons, *Baltimore County Panorama* (Towson, Md.: Baltimore County Public Library, 1988), pp. 203, 212. His father (1770–1833) designed an earlier four-story jail, engraved and labeled "Prison of Baltimore County & City" (finished 1800) on the border of T. H. Poppleton's *Plan of the City of Baltimore* (N.Y.: Harrison, 1823).

The extensive influence of Haviland's radial plan on prison architecture in the U.S. and especially abroad is described throughout Bruce Johnston et al., *Eastern State Penitentiary: Crucible of Good Intentions* (Philadelphia: Philadelphia Museum of Art, 1994), especially p. 105.

prevent double occupancy: a prisoner using the latrine was to carry with him a metal tag hanging by each door. This would enable the other prisoners on that floor to see that their latrine was occupied. Anyone leaving his place while the tag was gone from its hook was supposed to be severely punished.[52]

At this time, female prisoners, being fewer in number and also considered less unruly, were not subjected to the penitentiary discipline of silence and separation. Conversation among them was tolerated. They still slept in the congregate night rooms of the original west wing. Each room had five straw mattresses spread out on the floor, and the women slept two or three to a bed. But they were segregated from the men; during the day females worked in a separate building, engaged in spinning, knitting, and washing prison laundry. A wooden screen in the form of a venetian shutter ran along the western wall of their dormitory wing to prevent them from seeing men passing through the courtyard. And the men, in addition to being kept separate from the women, were now also segregated by race while they ate and worked.[53]

Even before construction of the new workshops had begun in May 1835, the Maryland Penitentiary had managed—since 1822—to improve greatly the productivity of its prison industries over the dismal performance of its first two decades.[54] Now, as the new radial workshops with their inspection corridors neared completion at the end of 1835, it was hoped that the institution could at last improve the discipline of male convicts in their workplace and bring about their moral reformation: "We confidently anticipate the most happy results," wrote General William McDonald, president of the board of directors of the penitentiary in their *Annual Report* (1836), "and therefore rejoice that it [the Auburn system] will soon be in full operation within this state."[55] But these great expectations were soon clouded by an investigation of the penitentiary that aired charges of lax discipline, mismanagement, and abuses of power.

---

[52]Demetz and Blouet, *Les pénitenciers des États Unis,* p. 37. All quotations from this work have been translated by the author.

[53]Ibid., pp. 37, 39 n.5. Before the completion of the new dormitory (1829) and workshops (1836), segregation of male prisoners by race was not practiced at the penitentiary. See the "Report of the Joint Committee Appointed to Visit the Penitentiary," *Journal of the House of Delegates* (1826), p. 425.

[54]Scharf, *History of Baltimore City and County,* p. 204.

[55]*Annual Report* (1836), p. 10.

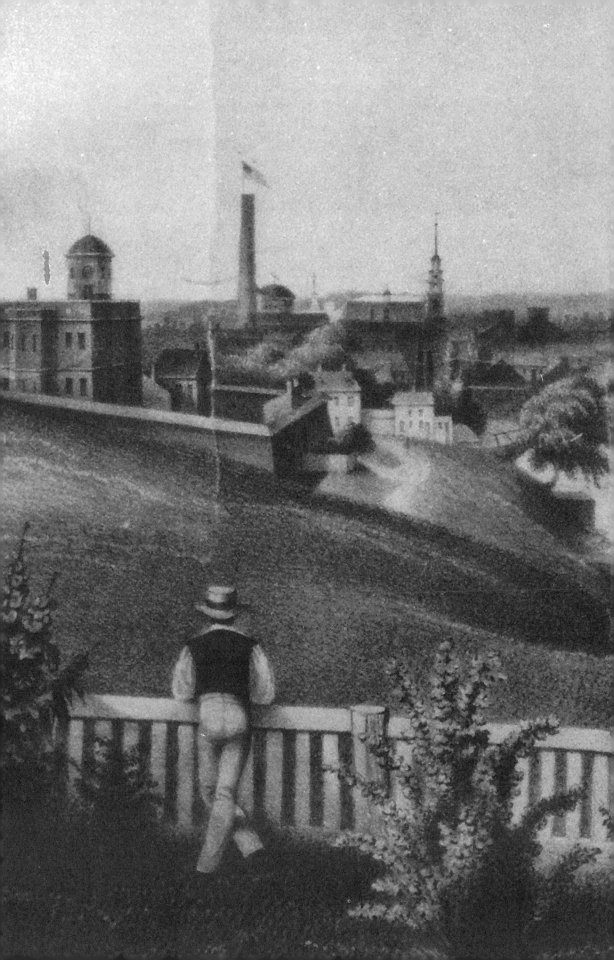

Chapter Two

The Investigation of 1837

Ironically, the very prosperity of the Maryland Penitentiary's industries generated political conflict both inside and outside its walls that for a time threatened the existence of the young institution. On February 5, 1836 and again on February 9, 1837, the "mechanics" of Baltimore City presented petitions to the Maryland House of Delegates to protest unfair competition from the prison's manufacturing departments, especially that of weaving.[1] On March 21, 1837, the legislature appointed a joint committee to investigate the affairs of the penitentiary and "particularly to enquire into the finance and police of the institution, and how far the several mechanical employments there prosecuted interfere with the mechanics of Baltimore."[2] The joint committee drew up a list of sixty-one multi-part questions to be answered orally or in writing by penitentiary officials, the first half concerning its management, the second almost exclusively about its weaving operations. The result was the first extensive published document in the penitentiary's history, a 430-page volume entitled *Testimony Taken before the Joint Committee of the Legislature on the Penitentiary* (1837).[3] From its pages emerges a bitter feud among penitentiary officials, who despite their personal animosities fought to keep the prison's lucrative weaving industry.

According to the written testimony of the penitentiary's board of directors, the weavers of Baltimore City had charged that cheap "criminal" labor enabled the institution to undersell textiles woven by "honest" citizens. The weavers wanted the legislature to halt this "injurious competition." In rebuttal the directors argued that when figuring the cost of convict labor, allowance must be made for those prisoners who contributed nothing directly to the financial support of the

---

[1]*Journal of the House of Delegates* (1834), p. 197, and (1836), p. 262.

[2]*Journal of the Senate* (1836), pp. 340–41.

[3]Hereafter cited as *Testimony.* The copy in the Maryland Room of the Enoch Pratt Free Library has on its title page the handwritten name of its original owner, Dr. H. Willis Baxley, a former medical officer and director of the penitentiary and one of the principal witnesses in the investigation.

Opposite: Detail from a lithograph of Baltimore made by Moses Swett and published in 1837, showing the Baltimore City Jail adjoining the western wall of the Maryland Penitentiary. (Maryland Historical Society.)

penitentiary: those too sick, infirm, or decrepit to work or those engaged in housekeeping chores. That meant the prisoners working at the 110 or 120 hand looms had to produce enough to cover the maintenance expenses of the other, non-productive prisoners. Figured this way, the directors said, the labor of convict weavers was actually more expensive than that of private factories. And because of this, the penitentiary had to obtain the highest market price for its goods in order to avoid becoming a burden on the state treasury. Contrary to being cheaper, said the directors, the prison-made textiles named in the complaint—linseys and cotton plaids and stripes—all sold "at much higher prices" than similar goods made by the city's weavers, and then added this rather unkind qualifier: "The Penitentiary goods are certainly . . . much better, and it is not to be denied that the best goods are generally the cheapest." The directors went on to say that the real competition for the city weavers came from the surrounding states, not from the penitentiary, whose share of the local market amounted to scarcely 1 percent; "at least three-fourths" of its textiles were sold to out-of-state traders. They concluded their rejoinder by saying that if prison industries were abolished, additional taxes would be required to support the penitentiary, and then idled prisoners would be denied all hope of reformation. Their testimony regarding the necessity of keeping prison industries, especially that of weaving, was supported—or at least not attacked—in the many pages of testimony given by all of the various penitentiary witnesses.[4]

But these same pages also revealed prolonged and nasty infighting among the penitentiary officials: on one side, Dr. H. Willis Baxley, a former medical officer and afterward a director, along with James McEvoy, who had served as clerk, treasurer, and secretary; on the other side, Warden Joseph Owens, along with the majority of the board of directors, including the board's powerful executive committee, composed of directors William H. Hanson and John G. Proud. The conflict apparently began over different priorities in managing the prison, with Dr. Baxley's side stressing the reformation of the convicts and Warden Owens's side their productivity. It then turned into a feud involving personal attacks, which are worth examining in some detail for the vivid picture given—rare for its time—of the penitentiary's day-to-day operations.

Dr. Baxley fired the opening shots in the published *Testimony,* accusing his erstwhile colleagues on the board of directors of failing to enforce the rules and regulations of the penitentiary and to impose the kind of discipline that would

---

[4] *Testimony,* pp. 30–33. Their testimony is too technical, statistical, and detailed to be summarized here and would be better suited for a more specialized economic history of the era, when power looms (used mainly by the weavers of Baltimore City) were gradually supplanting hand looms (the only kind used by the convict weavers).

bring about the moral reformation of the convicts. To support his charges he quoted recent observations about the penitentiary's lax discipline made by official visitors from foreign countries: Gustave de Beaumont and Alexis de Tocqueville from France (1833), William Crawford from England (1835), and Dr. Nicholas Julius from Prussia (1834). He then quoted the most recent visitor from France (identified only as "M. Devaux") who had inspected the new workshops and told him that "the State might wisely have saved the expense of their erection, if convicts, as he had seen, were allowed free access to the inspection avenues, (which he justly considered should be held as unapproachable precincts, and if the non-intercourse [silence] system were not rigidly enforced."[5]

Baxley then took aim at Warden Owens, listing his "illegal perquisites"—a house with convict servants and stable; fuel, candles, and oil; hogs fed with prison slops and cared for by convicts; and fruit, vegetable, and flower gardens tended by convict labor, the surplus products of which were sold for his family's benefit. Next came examples of the warden's allegedly poor discipline. According to Baxley, he allowed some convicts to keep their hair, contrary to the penitentiary regulation requiring their heads to be half-shaved (to discourage escapes). Three of these men subsequently escaped. He allowed the convict who looked after his stable to continue in his duties after being "detected in illicit intercourse with a female convict." A healthy but dangerous convict was permitted to stay in the hospital because he was making articles of dress for the warden's family. Another dangerous convict had custody of the keys to the punishment cells. The warden also encouraged prisoners to spy and inform on each other. Baxley then made a seemingly petty charge that assumed considerable importance in the later pages of the *Testimony*: that the warden had furnished prisoners with milk from his cows at full market price, even though the milk was skimmed and in warm weather often sour.[6]

When it came to matters of health, Dr. Baxley had much to say about the competence of the present penitentiary physician, Dr. Thomas B. Bond Jr. According to

---

[5] *Testimony*, pp. 103–4. I have been unable to find any published report in this country by "M. Devaux." The report of Beaumont and Tocqueville, on the other hand, was translated by Francis Lieber and published here: *On the Penitentiary System in the United States* (Philadelphia: Carey, Lea & Blanchard, 1833). The Englishman William Crawford's observations were published in *Report on the Penitentiaries of the United States* (1835), (reprinted Montclair, N.J.: Patterson Smith, 1969), pp. 94–101. Dr. Nicholas Julius published his observations in *Nordamerikas sittliche Zustände: Nach eigenen Anschauüngen in den Jahren 1834, 1835, und 1836*, 2 vols. (Leipzig: F. A. Brockhaus, 1839), noted by Johnston, *Eastern Penitentiary*, p. 109, n33.

The Maryland Penitentiary's tendency to subordinate reformation to productivity is also discussed by Marvin Gettleman, "The Maryland Penitentiary in the Age of Tocqueville, 1828–1842," *Maryland Historical Magazine*, 56 (1961): 286–90.

[6] *Testimony*, pp 105–6, 108–10. The inmate and the woman were caught together in a basement storeroom of the front (administration) building. Ironically, the man was named Charles Goodin, the woman nicknamed "Trusty." See testimony of James Disney, former deputy warden, in *Testimony*, p. 347.

Baxley, Bond had failed to state the facts regarding the accidental death of "coloured" prisoner Jacob Fountain by opium poisoning in November 1836. In December of the same year a supposedly insane convict had escaped from the hospital after deceiving Dr. Bond about his sanity, and another convict was pardoned by Bond, who, being a new physician, was unable to see how little a pardon was merited.[7]

Baxley's next target was the powerful two-man executive committee of the board of directors. This committee had grown in importance since it was first conceived. According to the penitentiary rules and regulations laid down in 1809, the twelve-man board of directors, or inspectors, as they were then called, met only every three months and therefore were to designate two of their number to visit the penitentiary at least once a week to oversee its management. By an act of 1826, this superintending committee was required to attend the penitentiary and its store-outlet for prison-made goods in the city three days a week, each member to receive two dollars for every day of attendance (the only directors to receive any compensation). A year later it was named the executive committee and was supposed to attend daily, if necessary. According to Baxley, the recent closing of the store-outlet for prison goods made daily visits unnecessary, and he alleged that the present members of the executive committee, William H. Hanson and John G. Proud, had illegally collected their two-dollar per diem each even when they had not visited the penitentiary. Believing that these men enjoyed a lucrative "sinecure" because of their membership on the board of directors, he recommended that the executive committee be abolished and replaced by a single person who was not a member of the board.[8]

Baxley also criticized the penitentiary's contract with director Thomas Kelso to furnish meat to the institution. Kelso, he alleged, manipulated his prices so as to discourage other suppliers from bidding and hence enjoyed a monopoly. Moreover, he said, the meat Kelso supplied was "unsound."[9]

Throughout these pages of his testimony, Baxley advocated strict discipline (no gambling, swearing, or use of tobacco) and close surveillance of the prisoners, not to punish but to reform them. He believed, for example, that the placement of the looms in the new workshops prevented the effective surveillance of the weavers and spoolers from the inspection avenues. His objections, he noted, were overruled by "those who look rather to manufacturing convenience [greater productivity] than to reformatory results."[10]

---

[7] *Testimony*, 110–20, 125. It appears that the prisoner Fountain was accidentally given three doses of paregoric by a male nurse in the hospital.

[8] *The Acts of Assembly; Together with the Governor's Proclamation and the Rules and Regulations Respecting the Penitentiary of Maryland* (Baltimore: J. Robinson, 1819), p. 28; *Testimony*, pp. 129–31.

[9] *Testimony*, pp. 133–35.

[10] Ibid., pp. 124, 136.

Baxley's testimony was followed by that of his ally, James McEvoy Jr., who had served as clerk—an important office, combining the duties of bookkeeper, treasurer, and secretary—at the penitentiary for ten years until his dismissal on April 21, 1836. McEvoy repeated Baxley's charge against the warden of lax discipline and accused the executive committee of frequent attempts to dominate him. Like Baxley, he believed the executive committee should be abolished and replaced by a single agent.[11]

As McEvoy described his struggles with the executive committee, the pages of the *Testimony* became truly rancorous. When a select committee of the legislature visited the penitentiary on January 26, 1836, and presented him with a list of questions regarding its general organization and administration, John G. Proud of the executive committee warned him not to submit his answers without first obtaining the approval of the board of directors. "Feeling indignant," McEvoy replied that he would not give any false statements or withhold any information from the special committee because of "any dread of the censorship of the directors" and that "no attempt had ever before been made to control the clerk in furnishing information." On February 16, after receiving the clerk's answers, the select committee introduced a bill to abolish the executive committee and appoint a single agent, other than a director, to perform their duties for $600 a year. According to McEvoy, the select committee's bill was the outcome of his "explicit and correct answers" to their questions and consequently provoked the board to take "a series of hostile measures" against him that ended with his dismissal.[12]

As related by McEvoy, the first hostile move occurred when executive committee member John G. Proud, in a breach of faith, told several members of the legislature that in the past the clerk had been charged with drinking intemperately. This piece of gossip had immediate repercussions. While Baxley was in Annapolis, General Ridgely of the House of Delegates asked him if the charge was true. Baxley admitted "that the clerk of the Penitentiary . . . would perhaps take a glass of wine or so too much sometimes, as other young men do, but that whoever should say he went further than that, would be guilty of a libel, a slander." When Baxley's remark reached his ears, Proud wrote him to say that he would not allow himself to be "considered a libeller, a slanderer, even by implication." The next day, Baxley wrote Proud a coldly threatening note asking if he

---

[11] *Testimony,* pp. 142–43, 146–47. He had succeeded his father, James McEvoy Sr., who had been clerk from at least 1816. See *Board of Directors Report,* 1816/17, p. 11.

[12] The clerk was specifically asked to describe the remaining duties of the executive committee after the recent closing of the penitentiary store freed them from supervising the sale of penitentiary goods there. *Report of the Select Committee of the Penitentiary to the Legislature of Maryland* (Annapolis, 1836), pp. 5–6. *Testimony,* pp. 154–57.

held himself "amenable to those laws ultimately appealed to by gentlemen in matters of personal difference [i.e., the code duello]." Proud did not reply.[13]

Next, according to McEvoy, on March 27 the president of the board of directors, General William McDonald, "with great warmth" reproached the clerk for his refusal to record in the minute book an earlier meeting of six directors—less than the legal quorum—to protest the bill to abolish the executive committee and said he would be "punished" by removal from office. Then on April 13 the executive committee, contrary to established procedure, bypassed the clerk and wrote their own formal notice to the commission merchants of Baltimore about a price increase in penitentiary cotton goods, knowing full well that the clerk would refuse to sign it. This was done, according to McEvoy, to arouse his indignation and to use his refusal to sign as one of the causes for his dismissal. Finally, on April 21 the clerk was removed from office by a seven-to-five vote of the board of directors. No charges were made at the time, though the removing party were challenged to do so.[14]

As McEvoy continued, he laid bare what he took to be a source of the executive committee's power. The clerk testified that warden Owens had earnestly opposed the existence of the executive committee for nine years preceding John G. Proud's appointment to it in the summer of 1835, after which time he became one of its earnest supporters. "There can be no reason for Mr. O's present (or recent) support of the committee," said McEvoy, "other than the circumstance that Mr. Proud is an intimate friend and adviser of Mr. N. F. Williams, a member of the [Governor's] executive council, to whom Mr. O. looks for his own appointment."[15]

Like his ally Dr. Baxley, the clerk believed in the importance of prison discipline for the reformation of the convicts. In his eyes the bill to abolish the executive committee was crucial to the success of the penitentiary as an institution to reform the criminals in its care. The new workshops were well adapted for the "admirable" Auburn system of discipline, he said, but this potential could not be realized until the entire board of directors took control of the penitentiary's operation. "At present," he said, "half of them . . . [are] willing instruments of the executive committee." Until the board lived up to its responsibilities, he went on to say, "the Maryland Penitentiary will continue to

---

[13] The charge was made in a report by the executive committee to the board of directors on November 18, 1835. It was settled in a hearing by three directors: McEvoy was pardoned for his lapse and the matter kept secret on the condition he would not repeat his offense. McEvoy claimed to have kept his pledge. *Testimony,* pp. 180–83.

[14] Ibid., pp. 174–77.

[15] Ibid., pp. 177–78.

be, as it has been, a manufacturing establishment alone," without fulfilling its other goal of reforming the convicts.[16]

Still other bits of political intrigue were revealed in McEvoy's closing testimony: he reproached a new member of the board of directors, the Reverend Thomas Bond, for having "united with the other directors in assigning false reasons for the clerk's removal." Here one can guess the Reverend Mr. Bond's motive for opposing McEvoy: he was the father of Dr. Thomas Bond Jr., the current penitentiary physician, whose competence had been attacked by the clerk's ally, Baxley. Finally the clerk testified that the executive committee had renewed the penitentiary's annual beef contract with another director, Thomas Kelso, despite McEvoy's protest over its "exorbitant" price.[17]

The reply of Warden Joseph Owens to Dr. Baxley's charge took up only several pages and consisted mostly of simple denials. As for the charge against him of selling sour milk to the hospital, Owens said that no complaint had ever been made and added this innuendo: "if there was any sour milk found in the hospital by Dr. Baxley, it was made so by being kept there during the night, to make cream for the Doctor's breakfast in the morning, which meal for many months he was in the habit of taking in the hospital department, although there never had been any perquisites attached to his office."[18]

In contrast to Warden Owens, penitentiary physician Thomas Bond Jr. delivered a tirade against Baxley, who he said had shown "all the malignity of the devil without the apology of revenge; . . . since the arch-fiend villified poor Job before the angels, I know of no one who has taken more pains to rummage after charges made against individuals, hitherto unsuspected." He then gave a long and technically detailed defense of his conduct in connection with the death of the "coloured" prisoner, Jacob Fountain, from opium poisoning, a case which he described as "the penitentiary comedy in which the Doctor [Baxley] has figured with such unenvied applause."[19]

When his turn came again, Baxley cited chapter and verse of Owens's testimony in a long and tenacious rebuttal, during which he renewed his charge against the warden of purveying sour milk. Baxley said his complaints about it led to an inquiry by the board of directors, with the result that the penitentiary bought cows to furnish its own supply of milk to the hospital. Because of this loss of profit, said Baxley, the warden "fastened on me his unforgiving hatred, and has exposed me to an untiring persecution." He went on to deny any illegal

---

[16]Ibid., pp. 178–79.
[17]Ibid., p. 184.
[18]Ibid., pp. 185–87.
[19]Ibid., p. 188.

perquisite by breakfasting at the hospital: it was provided by the matron of the prison at her expense "in consideration of my professional services given to herself and her family."[20]

Turning once more to Dr. Bond, Baxley complained of his "petulant abuse and personal hatred" and then said that his appointment as penitentiary physician along with his father's as a director were proposed by a member of the executive committee (unnamed, but probably John G. Proud) to create a faction. The partisan directors voted in favor of the proposals and thereby "established a community of interest which made them the reciprocal supporters of each other's wishes."[21] Like McEvoy, Baxley believed that a tangled web of political alliances among the board of directors, its executive committee, and the warden stood in the way of a clean and efficient administration of the penitentiary.

Once the principals in the penitentiary feud had had their say, other witnesses came forward with testimony alleging lax discipline, shady practices, or abuses of power on the part of Warden Joseph Owens. Chief among them was James Disney, a former deputy warden until his removal from office by the board of directors in March 1834. Disney gave an example of favoritism practiced by Owens. Most convicts ate ordinary prison fare in the refectory in the morning and at noon and were given a piece of bread at the day's end to take with them into their cells. But certain prisoners—the gardener, tailor, barber, and bootblack—were sent such leftovers from the warden's table as pies, cold ham, and chicken. Moreover, the convicts were not kept separate after work, he said, but had many chances to form "combinations," i.e., cliques or gangs. "They sat about in the yard in crowds . . . consulting their own wishes as to what they should do." Also, according to Disney, Warden Owens used informers, and unreliable ones at that. A certain convict was supposed to give warning of an intended escape. When the prisoners did make their attempt, the informer, William Low, proved to be the "the greatest rascal among them, and a dictator and leader in the insurrection." He was subsequently pardoned out and since then had been convicted on the charge of stealing.[22]

Disney's testimony regarding lax discipline was backed up by former guard John Demuth, who said the convicts were not hindered from talking together in the old workshops. "The privy was a common place where they resorted." And he repeated the charge of illegal perquisites made earlier by Dr. Baxley: Warden Owens used convict labor to raise hogs, chickens, vegetables, and flowers for his own use.[23]

---

[20]Ibid., pp. 281–96.
[21]Ibid., pp. 297–99.
[22]Ibid., pp. 216–20, 348.
[23]Ibid., p. 224.

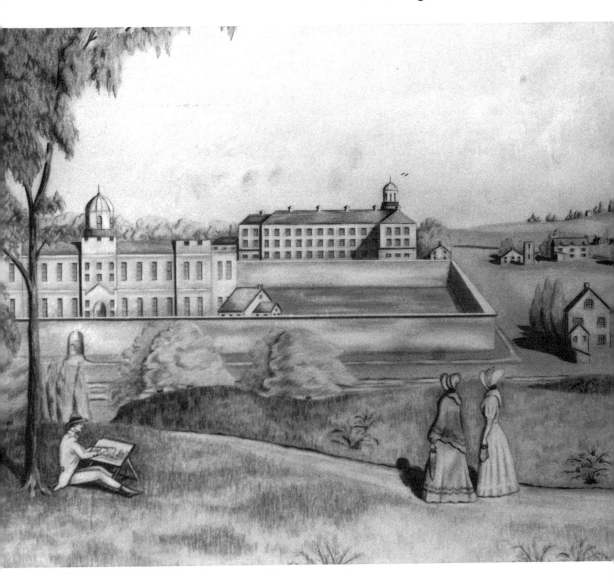

This idealized sketch (1837) shows the City Jail (left) enclosed by walls and the penitentiary's first dormitory (center), beyond which rises the cupola of its administration building. The three-acre site near the Jones Falls had been carefully chosen by a legislative commission because it was "high and elevated, commanding an extensive and interesting prospect, and which must always enjoy a free circulation of air from its altitude over the surrounding ground" (*Maryland Penitentiary Penal Commission Report*, 1913).

Yet another questionable dealing by the warden surfaced towards the end of the *Testimony* when former penitentiary physician Dr. James Reardan[24] submitted a copy of the will made by a dying prisoner, dated August 24, 1834. Frederick Clause had entered the hospital on a Friday with a strangulated hernia and died the following Sunday. In his will, signed that same day, he left a large tract of land (289 acres) in Allegany County, Maryland, and his whole estate to his "worthy and best friend, Mr. Joseph Owens" and named Owens his executor.[25]

Having read over the allegations of abuses made by Baxley and his party to the investigating committee, the board wrote a separate defense in a fourteen-page "Reply of the Directors to the Charges Against the Penitentiary,"[26] addressed to the chairman, Israel D. Maulsby. These allegations, according to the "Reply," originated in a personal quarrel between Warden Owens and Dr. Baxley while the latter was penitentiary physician in 1833. When Baxley was appointed a director in 1835, he tried to have Owens removed from office, being aided by his personal friends, the clerk (McEvoy) and the new physician (Reardan). When the directors did not reappoint his two friends upon the expiration of their terms, Baxley approached a visiting legislative committee and instigated the present full-scale investigation of the penitentiary's management.[27]

The board then tartly replied to charges made against them and the warden by their accusers. Among them: if Baxley believed that discipline was lax or that the warden behaved improperly, they said, he could have brought these matters to the board's notice while he himself was a member in the two years (1835–36) preceding the investigation—but he did not. Regarding the warden's alleged perquisite of a vegetable garden: no such garden had existed within the walls of the penitentiary for several years. The charge exemplified the "utter recklessness" of Baxley's allegations against penitentiary authorities. As to the purchase of supplies for the penitentiary from several directors: there was no law against it, and besides, Baxley's own father once sold drugs and medicines to the institution "for a considerable period." And McEvoy's complaint about his drinking problem being made public knowledge came about because Baxley "surreptitiously" obtained the sealed packet containing a committee report of same ("a gross impropriety approaching to moral turpitude, in the conduct of Dr. H. Willis Baxley") and gave it to McEvoy, who foolishly gave it to the investigating committee as evidence of his supposed harassment. Their "Reply" closed

---

[24]Reardan lost his post along with the clerk, James McEvoy, because he opposed the warden and the executive committee. See the testimony of former director William Jenkins, *Testimony,* p. 99.

[25]Ibid., pp. 382–83.

[26]Baltimore: Printed by J. W. Woods, 1837. Appended to *Board of Directors Report* (1838).

[27]*Testimony,* pp. 3–4.

with disdainful references to McEvoy's "various falsehoods and misrepresentations" and to the "hearsay" evidence of one James H. Raymond, who had written accusations against them in a newspaper for "political effect."[28]

When the *Testimony* was published, it did not contain the findings of the investigative joint committee, which were presented to the legislature on January 20, 1838.[29] In their report, the joint committee exonerated the penitentiary administration of underselling the textiles made by the weavers of Baltimore. They agreed with the argument of the board of directors that the penitentiary was forced to sell its goods at the highest, not the lowest prices, to cover the maintenance of non-productive prisoners and hence did not compete unfairly. Using strong language, the joint committee declared themselves satisfied "that the abandonment of manufacturing in the penitentiary would be equivalent to a destruction of the institution, for without carrying on manufactures, it could not be supported except by the Treasury of the State." The committee then added this comment about the reformative value of prison labor: "Coercive punishment is of little use, unless criminals are rendered virtuous by discipline."[30]

But the committee's report was critical of the penitentiary's administration and proposed numerous changes in its appended "Act relating to the Maryland Penitentiary," most of them arising from the charges made by Baxley and McEvoy. It found the executive committee insufficiently accountable because, being made up of board members, they could vote on and control their actions. As a remedy, the joint committee proposed the replacement of the executive committee by two agents not connected with the penitentiary and appointed by the governor. Moreover, the report said that the executive committee's daily visits to the penitentiary were presumed by the board of directors to make additional visits by themselves unnecessary, with the unintended result that the administration of prison discipline and commercial activity had been left up to the warden and the executive committee, respectively. The report also found that the board of directors had too many members to function effectively and proposed a reduction from twelve members to six, a number nearer to that of other prison boards.[31]

The report then focused on certain "irregularities" committed by individual officials. It found "improper" Warden John Owens's practice of sending occasional "delicacies" to certain convicts. It declared illegal his use of convicts as

---

[28]Ibid., pp. 5–6, 9, 13, 15–16.

[29]"Report of the Joint-Committee Appointed by the General Assembly to Investigate the Affairs of the Maryland Penitentiary," printed as an appendix to the *Journal of Proceedings of the Senate of Maryland* (December session, 1837).

[30]*Testimony,* pp. 75–96.

[31]Ibid., pp. 25–27.

servants, even though sanctioned by the board of directors, and said it had led "to improper intercourse among the convicts." It deplored the "system of espionage." With reference to the dying convict's will which left his whole estate to the warden, the report pronounced the warden's acceptance of this gift as "wholly inadmissible." Also, without actually naming Thomas Kelso, it condemned his contract to supply the penitentiary with beef and recommended a law prohibiting any director or officer from selling any article of provision whatsoever to the penitentiary.[32]

But though critical of the penitentiary's management, the investigating committee throughout its report seemed anxious to avoid the kind of outright condemnation that might bring down its whole administration and threaten the existence of the young institution. They apologized for including in the published *Testimony* "the exhibition of personal animosity, and indulgence in offensive language" but said it was the inevitable admixture in the testimony of witnesses who had personal differences. The committee expressed obligation to all parties who cooperated in the investigation, adding that it should not be supposed that "your committee intend to censure the directors and officers by making suggestions at variance with some of the practices observed at the house." They had found no purposeful mismanagement, they said, or any desire to frustrate the prosperity of the penitentiary. Far from heaping blame on the penitentiary's administrators, they closed on a conciliatory note: "We anticipate that under their management and direction, with the changes recommended by us, the penitentiary cannot fail to produce the most salutary and lasting benefits to the people of the State."[33]

The board of directors, however, would not be bought off by the conciliatory language that ended the joint committee's report and made a last attempt to protect their turf. In February 1838, barely a month after the committee had presented its report, the board sent the General Assembly a long "Memorial" (also appended to their annual report for 1838) vigorously protesting nearly all the changes proposed by the committee in the "Act relating to the Maryland Penitentiary." Among them: the reduction of the number of directors from twelve to six and the abolishment of its executive committee. After two veiled but unmistakable references to the hostile testimony of former director Baxley, clerk McEvoy, and former penitentiary physician Reardan, the directors closed by saying that their situation had lately been made "almost intolerable" by politically motivated accusations in the newspapers. They described their own expe-

---

[32]Ibid., pp. 28–31.

[33]Ibid., pp. 101–2. The joint committee's report also contains many pages of statistics regarding the penitentiary's finances and manufacturing that cannot be included in this historical essay.

rience during the recent investigation as a "fiery ordeal" and ended by offering to resign. "The storm having passed, they are ready to make a place for others, if any are desirous to have them. . . . and having given their views, will most cheerfully abide the action of the General Assembly."[34]

Exactly what action, if any, was taken by the General Assembly is not clear 150 years later. But the apparent winners of the bitter feud are to be seen in the roster of penitentiary officials in the next surviving annual report (1839), which shows the reappointment of Dr. H. Willis Baxley to the board of directors, now numbering only six, and James McEvoy as clerk. The executive committee was abolished, and the names of the other directors and of the warden were all new. The administration had been both streamlined and cleaned up. The young institution had survived its first political storm.

---

[34] *Testimony,* pp. 22, 24, 28–29.

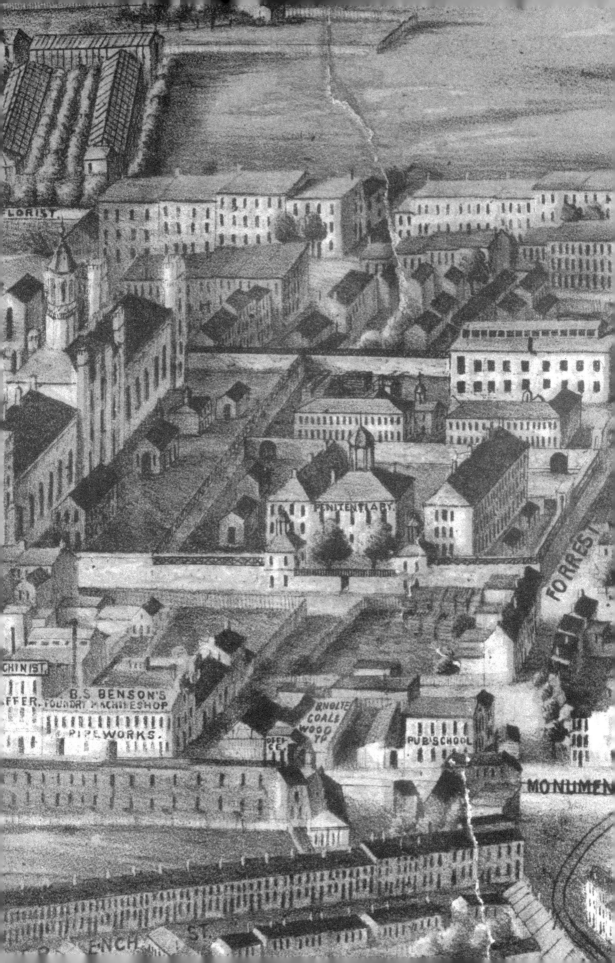

Chapter Three

New Ways in Penology

1838 – 1888

The bitter feud among the penitentiary officials had ended with the departure of the losing faction. Now, without the distractions of cronyism and petty bickering among its staff, the young institution could once more focus its attention on its two main goals—to support itself through the productive labor of its inmates and to bring about their moral reformation. For the next half-century of relative harmony in its administration, the penitentiary would prove receptive to innovative practices at other prisons and to fresh theories or ideas of such prison reformers as Louis Dwight, Francis Lieber, Dorothea Dix, and Enoch C. Wines.[1]

But first the financial health of the institution became an immediate and pressing concern because its very existence could be threatened if it continued to burden taxpayers.[2] Although the legislature had allowed the penitentiary to keep its heretofore lucrative hand-loom industry, the nation's mercantile crisis of 1837 ended the long period of prosperity previously enjoyed by all the prison's industries. Profits from the penitentiary's cotton and woolen goods fell partly because of a decrease in demand for those goods and partly because of competition from labor-saving machinery. Yet another contributing cause was that the prison labor pool had shrunk, "a result in part of the law of 1836, ordering that negroes, upon re-conviction of crime, be sold out of the State." From 1837 to 1841 inclusive, the deficit amounted to $46,683.17.[3]

---

[1]Blake McKelvey, *American Prisons: A History of Good Intentions* (Montclair, N.J.: Patterson Smith, 1977), p. 35.

[2]The young institution had its skeptics in the state legislature as recently as 1822, when a special committee there recommended the abolishment of the penitentiary if it could not do better at reforming its inmates and supporting itself financially through their labor. See *Journal of the House of Delegates* (1822), pp. 139–40.

[3]*Report of the Committee on Prison Manufactures, Maryland Penitentiary* (Baltimore: Lucas & Deaver, 1842), pp. 3–6, and "A Sketch of the Maryland Penitentiary, Its Origin and Progress," appended to the *Board of Directors Report* (1881), p. 56.

Opposite: The Maryland State Penitentiary as presented in E. Sachse & Co.'s *Bird's Eye View of the City of Baltimore, 1869,* a year before construction of "C" dormitory. (Maryland Historical Society.)

The penitentiary searched for ways to staunch this flow of red ink. First it tried to establish the manufacture of more profitable goods than cotton and woolen textiles. In 1841 it set up a trial shoe operation, which for a while looked promising. Two years later it bought special looms and tried manufacturing fancy silk goods, which for several years proved very profitable, but swift changes in fashion turned the financial experiment into a disaster. Meanwhile, in 1847 the penitentiary was forced to stop its once profitable operation of sawing stone by hand because it could not compete with establishments using steam-powered saws. Its final experiment, toward the end of the decade, was to set a few prisoners to work making wrought nails.[4]

While these futile experiments with new products were being carried on, the penitentiary also considered changing its current way of using convict labor. From its very beginning, the prison had managed its workshop industries directly under what became known as the state account system. The prison bought the materials, provided the necessary tools or machinery, supervised its workers, and handled the sales of its products—through a prison outlet store in Baltimore before 1833, and afterwards through commission houses charging 6 percent.[5] Under this system, the prosperity of the penitentiary's industries naturally depended on general trade conditions. The alternate way was to hire out its convict labor to a private entrepreneur under the so-called contract system, in which the contractor provided the materials and paid the prison a fixed rate per day per man for his labor. Under this system, the prosperity of the penitentiary was less vulnerable to fluctuating trade conditions.

The contract system had been suggested as early as 1825 by the legislature.[6] It was actually given a trial at the penitentiary in July 1833, according to the board of directors' *Report* for that year. Forty convicts were set to work hammering granite under the supervision of a contractor, who paid the penitentiary fifty cents a day per man. Whether the contractor worked the prisoners too hard cannot be proven, but the same report contained this suggestive passage: "Several instances have occurred among the convicts of their having deliberately and wilfully maimed themselves by inflicting severe wounds, or by cutting off their fingers, so as to become incapable of performing useful labor." Furthermore, on the night of February 18, 1834, the granite sheds were destroyed by fire, and arson was suspected.[7]

---

[4]*Board of Directors Report* (1841), p. 5, and supplement to the *Board of Directors Report* (1848), pp. 3–4.

[5]Marvin Gettleman, "The Maryland Penitentiary in the Age of Tocqueville, 1828–1842," *Maryland Historical Magazine,* 56 (1961): 289, n3.

[6]*Journal of the House of Delegates of Maryland,* December Session, 1825, p. 77. Noted by Gettleman, p. 288, n73.

[7]*Board of Directors Report* (1834), pp. 3–6, 10.

In 1842 the penitentiary's specially appointed Committee on Prison Manufactures journeyed north to inspect certain state prisons (New York, Connecticut, and Massachusetts) where the contract system was being used. At that time, the committee found the contract system not suited to the Maryland Penitentiary mainly because the low rate the contractor paid for prison labor meant that it would compete with that of free workers. The resulting public outcry would threaten the very existence of the penitentiary system. This had been the case, the committee said, especially in New York, "where a wish is even to some extent prevalent, to abolish prisons and revert to the former modes of employing the convicts upon roads and other public works." In 1848 the penitentiary's directors further objected to the contract system because it seemed no more profitable than the one currently in use and because it could endanger the reformation of the prisoners, given the natural tendency of the contractor to extract as much work as he could from them.[8]

But the penitentiary's shaky financial condition made it necessary to give the contract system another trial. When a select committee of the legislature visited the penitentiary in 1852, it reported favorably on current experiments with contract labor. The directors had employed almost fifty convicts in making spikes and had farmed out another group making brooms with good results. In 1855 the directors sent yet another committee north to observe the operation of the contract system in leading prisons. On the basis of a favorable report, the directors expanded their use of the contract system by hiring out the labor of a hundred hands from their own manufacturing operations for the following year. But the penitentiary's overall financial condition deteriorated in 1857, first because of the economic depression, which "disturbed the credit of the whole civilized world." To worsen matters, a fire destroyed the north wing of the workshops, throwing two hundred hands out of work for five months. More was to come. Four years later, the directors reported that their high hopes for the financial recovery of the institution had been blighted by "the distressing calamity of civil war," and that in one year the income from contract labor had dropped from $35,000 to $7,800. Despite these interruptions, the contract labor system had by now become established at the Maryland Penitentiary and in time would provide the basis for its second period of great prosperity, from 1872 to 1881.[9]

----

[8]*Report of the Committee on Prison Manufactures* (1842), p. 13; Supplement to the *Board of Directors Report* (1848), p. 5.

[9]*Board of Directors Report* (1857), pp. 3, 5; "Sketch of the Maryland Penitentiary," in *Board of Directors Report* (1881), pp. 75–78, 80–82, 60–61, and 65–68; and Thomas Wilkinson, "The Maryland Penitentiary," in J. Thomas Scharf, *History of Baltimore City and County from the Earliest Period to the Present Day* (1881), p. 204.

Overleaf: The City of Baltimore, 1855, by Joseph Hutchins Colton, graphically shows the extent to which the city had expanded to surround the penitentiary by mid-century. Collection of Willard Hackerman.

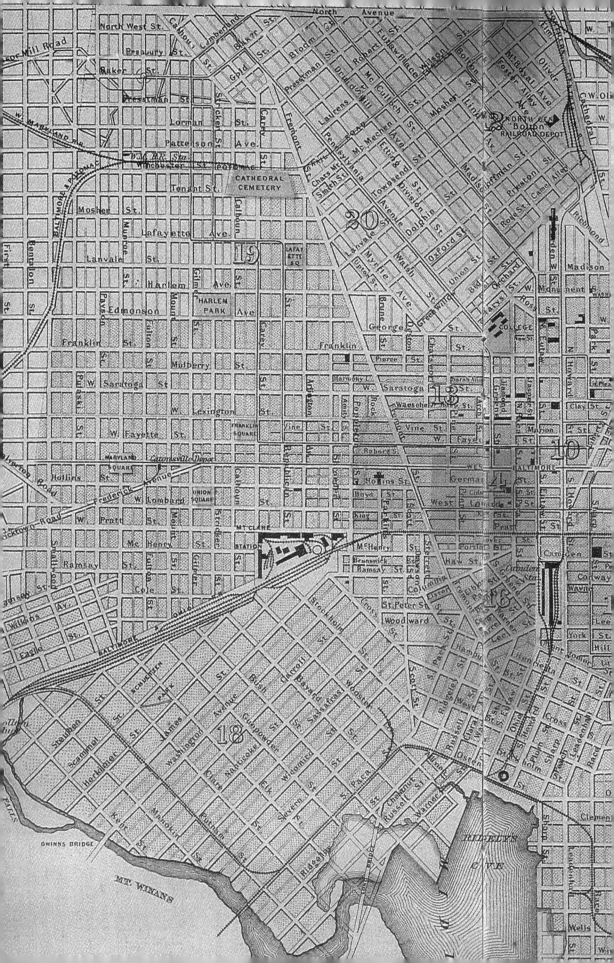

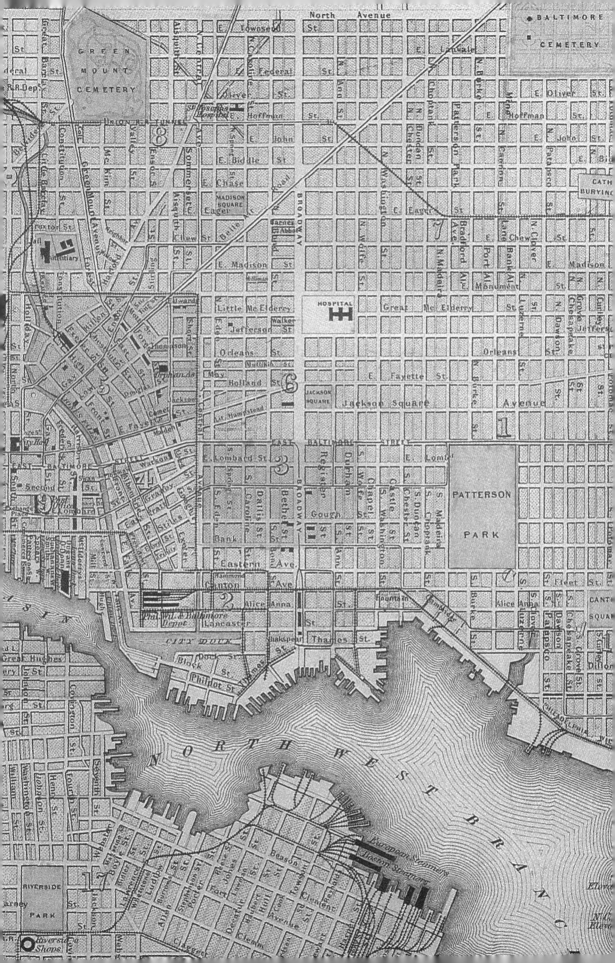

Not all the blame for the penitentiary's financial troubles could be ascribed to the state account system, whose prosperity was so directly linked to general trade conditions. A penurious state legislature doled out money to the prison at irregular intervals and in quantities that never allowed the institution enough operating capital for unforeseen contingencies or fluctuating trade conditions. As a result, the penitentiary was forced at times to sell its goods at unfavorable prices in order to raise cash to pay the salaries of its officers and buy supplies and materials. On other occasions it had to borrow the necessary money and pay out large sums of interest. "Figuratively speaking," reported the directors in 1850, "the manufacturers of the Maryland Penitentiary are constantly in a pawn broker's shop."[10]

Yet another drag on the institution's balance sheet was the policy of sending petty offenders to the penitentiary for relatively short prison terms, some for as little as three to six months but the majority from eighteen months to three years. Because six to twelve months of training were required before a convict became truly productive in a prison industry, the directors observed in 1848, "he is most likely [to be] discharged, his term having expired, just when his labor is beginning to be profitable to the institution." This particular problem would not be solved until 1878, when the new House of Correction opened its doors to receive petty offenders.[11]

Although the penitentiary administration relentlessly sought ways to become financially self-supporting, it never abandoned its other main goal—the moral reformation of its convicts. Prison industry was supposed to further this aim through the cultivation of regular habits of work and thrift, an idea publicly expressed by such prison reformers as Francis Wayland, Francis Lieber, and the highly influential Reverend Louis Dwight, founder of the Boston Prison Discipline Society.[12] However, in the eyes of prison officials, the larger problem posed by the Auburn penal system (congregate work in silence during the day, confinement in separate cells at night) was to keep the prisoners from hatching plots and otherwise socially corrupting each other while at work.

The Maryland Penitentiary's new radial workshops with their inspection avenues down the center allowed for better surveillance of the working prisoners. In common with other institutions using the Auburn system, the penitentiary enforced the rule of silence and attention to work with the lash. But in 1839 the largely new board of directors (Dr. H. Willis Baxley had been reinstated) showed a willingness to experiment with more humane methods of dis-

---

[10]"A Sketch of the Maryland Penitentiary," in *Board of Directors Report* (1881), p. 56.

[11]Supplement to the *Board of Directors Report* (1848), p. 6. See also "A Sketch of the Maryland Penitentiary," in *Board of Directors Report* (1881), pp. 62, 85–86.

[12]Gettleman, "The Maryland Penitentiary in the Age of Tocqueville," p. 288, and McKelvey, *American Prisons*, pp. 15–16.

cipline. Proudly they announced that "corporal punishment has been greatly mitigated in its rigor by the adoption of an instrument for the purpose, inflicting a degree of pain, more transient in duration and of much less severity than that which was caused by the implement [the lash] formerly in use."[13] They did not name the new instrument, but quite possibly it was the cold shower bath, which was being tried at various prisons[14] during this time. The punishment records of the penitentiary published in the 1847 *Board of Directors Report* show that twenty-seven shower baths had been given, chiefly to female offenders; "stripes" were still the standard punishment for male convicts and had reached a peak in 1843 during the harsh tenure of Warden A. I. W. Jackson (1842–45). In that year 9,527 stripes were given to only 290 male prisoners, an average of thirty-three per man.[15]

Upon the departure of Warden Jackson in 1845, efforts were made by various enlightened wardens to reduce the number of stripes dealt out to male offenders. His successor, Warden William Johnson (1845–48), in 1846 lowered the number of stripes to 2,482, or about one-quarter of the peak level. He was succeeded by Warden Isaac Denson (1848–51), who reduced this number further to six hundred. Denson accomplished this, he said, "by substituting deprivation of meals . . . so much less revolting to humanity, so much less degrading to offenders."[16]

Though there is no firm evidence for it, this mitigation of severe punishment may have owed something to the recent visits to the penitentiary by that redoubtable prison reformer, Dorothea Dix. While gathering information on prisons in the eastern United States, Miss Dix visited the Maryland Penitentiary twice in 1845, the last visit in July. Later that same year she published her brief but influential book, *Remarks on Prisons and Prison Discipline in the United States*. Here she conceded the necessity of using the lash for the most refractory prisoners but preferred the shower bath and went on to say: "I think most prisoners would yield as readily to a shower procured by a single bucket of water, as by a dozen lashes: the lash hardens a hard nature, and degrades a degraded one."[17]

Another enlightened warden who preferred the carrot to the stick to encourage good conduct was John W. Horn (1867–72, 1882–88), whose policies seem to have been directly influenced by the *Report of the Prisons and Reformatories of the*

---

[13]*Board of Directors Report* (1839), p. 8.

[14]According to Dorothea Dix's *Remarks on Prisons and Prison Discipline in the United States* (1845), the cold shower had been tried at prisons in Trenton, N.J., Columbus, Ohio, and Auburn and Sing Sing, N.Y. (pp. 14, 17, 19, 24).

[15]*Board of Directors Report* (1847), pp. 13–14.

[16]*Board of Directors Report* (1849), pp. 14–15.

[17]*Remarks on Prisons and Prison Discipline in the United States* (1845; repr. Montclair, N.J.: Patterson Smith, 1967), pp. 24–25. The 1845 *Board of Directors Report* noted: "a number of works [not named] received

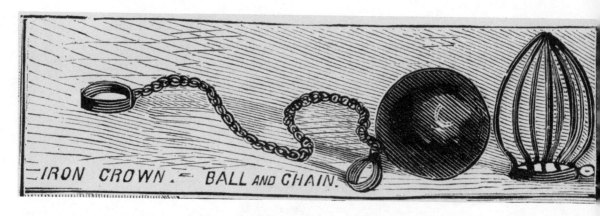

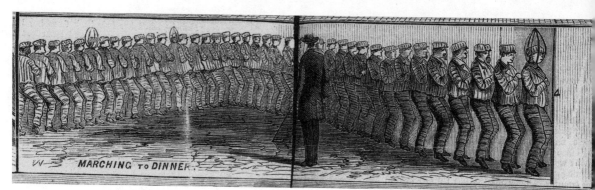

Above: Two nineteenth-century punishments employed in penitentiaries around the country. At the penitentiary at Ossining, New York, three of the prisoners marching in lockstep to dinner wear the cruel iron cap or crown, an almost medieval device never used at the Maryland Penitentiary. The more common ball and chain was designed to humiliate as well as hinder. It was last used at the Maryland Penitentiary in 1920.

Opposite: Many institutions regarded the cold shower bath, shown in use at Sing-Sing, as an effective corporal punishment and more humane than the lash. The Maryland Penitentiary was among the earliest prisons to use it, experimentally, in the 1840s. (*Harper's Weekly,* June 22, 1867. Enoch Pratt Free Library, Baltimore.)

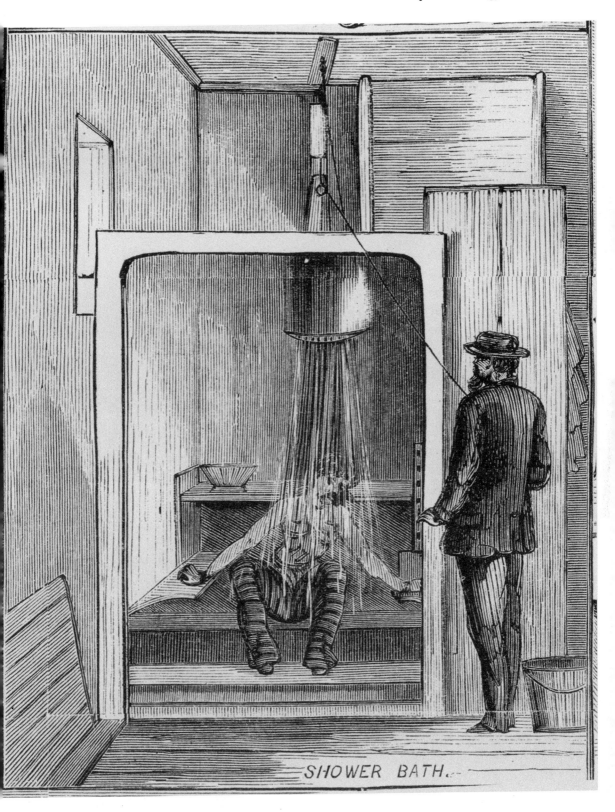

SHOWER BATH.

United States and Canada, written in 1867 by Enoch C. Wines and Theodore Dwight. In this landmark of penological reform, Wines and Dwight noted that nine states had already passed commutation laws (providing time off for good behavior) and quoted various prison officials on the beneficial results, including a memorable one from P. T. Miller of the Missouri state penitentiary: "As a disciplinary measure, this [commutation] law is worth all the shower-baths, dark cells, iron caps, lashes, bucks, crucifixes, and other refined methods of punishment, known to the science of penology."[18] Wines and Dwight then reported that Miller had tried to relieve the monotony of prison life by allowing the inmates to amuse themselves on public holidays (the Fourth of July, Thanksgiving, and Christmas) with theatrical performances, special meals, and athletics. Warden Horn appears to have adopted these reforms as his own. In the 1867 *Annual Report,* he urged the passage of Maryland's version of commutation—the "good time law"—noting its recent adoption by several other states and expressing his belief that such policy would "forever abolish the lash."[19] Two years later the penitentiary directors referred in their *Report* to Warden Horn's humanity, saying that the lash had been almost abolished for trivial offenses in favor of confinement to cell or the wearing of the ball and chain. They also said that more free time had been granted prisoners as well as such privileges as exercise, entertainment, and holidays.[20]

Not all these reforms lasted, however, because discipline—including the lock-step and rule of silence—was maintained by different prison officials as they saw fit within limitations imposed by the penitentiary's *Rules and Regulations* (1871), which still allowed the warden to punish offenders with up to thirteen stripes and ten days on bread and water.[21] Though female offenders in

---

from Miss Dix" (p. 7). As for the personal qualities of Miss Dix, Helen E. Marshall refers to her as being stubborn and headstrong and says: "Dorothea Dix would always have her way in life." See Helen E. Marshall, *Dorothea Dix: Forgotten Samaritan* (Chapel Hill: University of North Carolina Press, 1937), p. 17.

[18]The *iron cap,* or *crown* was worn by the offender day and night and interfered with normal eating, drinking, and sleep as well as being a visible sign of degradation to his fellow prisoners. The *buck* was like a large sawbuck or sawhorse. The offender was made to sit astride its narrow rail or beam for an extended period without his feet touching the ground. The *crucifix* was a large horizontal wooden cross upon which the offender (usually violent) was tied down as a forcible restraint.

[19]*Report of the Prisons and Reformatories of the United States and Canada* (Albany, N.Y.: Van Benthuysen & Sons' Steam Printing House, 1867; repr. New York: AMS Press, 1973), pp. 153–56, 157, 159, 161. Maryland did not pass the "good time law" until 1876. See *Board of Directors Report* (1876), p. 4.

[20]While discussing the new freedoms allowed blacks in the half-dozen years following the Civil War, Sherry Olson writes, "Even in the penitentiary the black prisoners celebrated the Fourth by making ice cream, parading with fife and drum, playing baseball, and performing plantation jigs." See Olson, *Baltimore: the Building of an American City* (Baltimore: Johns Hopkins University Press, 1980), p. 188.

[21]Male prisoners were whipped at the penitentiary until 1905/6, when the practice was discontinued by Warden John F. Weyler for sanitary reasons. Weyler believed the blood-soaked cat-o'-nine-tails could transmit syphilis when used on the next offender. See *Report of the Maryland Penitentiary Penal Commission* (1913), pp. 49–50.

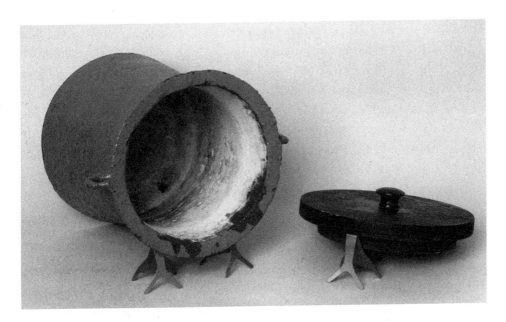

A "filth bucket," used throughout the nineteenth century in the prison's dungeon-like cells. In 1899 the penitentiary constructed new cellblocks of steel, each cell having a combination lavatory and flush toilet. (Photograph by Alan Scherr. Courtesy of the Maryland Division of Correction.)

the 1840s had been subjected to the experimental punishment of the cold showerbath, the lash continued to be used on them regularly. A sample page from the last surviving punishment ledger of the penitentiary for this period shows that as late as August 1878 (Warden Thomas S. Wilkinson), Mary Cassidy and Rachel Johnson each received five stripes for "Cursing, quarreling and fighting," and in September, Hennie Harrison and Fannie Blair each received five stripes for "Indecent conduct." Thereafter in these pages the punishment of stripes for female convicts becomes less frequent, perhaps because of public opinion or because of a growing reluctance on the part of penitentiary officials to inflict such severe corporal punishment on women.[22]

Besides these attempts to mitigate severe corporal punishment, other penal reforms or experiments in rehabilitation were considered or tried throughout this period. In their 1846 *Report,* the penitentiary directors noted that insane

[22]"Rules Violation Records — Females" (1873–89), p. 19. Maryland Historical Records #5666, Maryland State Archives. It is possible, however, that sporadic whipping of female convicts lasted into the next century, though there is no firm evidence for it. During its investigation of the penitentiary in 1913, the Maryland Penitentiary Penal Commission had heard convict testimony "tending to prove that both white and colored women had been stripped to the waist and whipped with the cat." The commission then questioned warden emeritus John F. Weyler (1888–1912) about this charge and received this equivocal answer: "I would be positive that I did not whip any white woman in the last ten years." See *Report of the Maryland Penitentiary Penal Commission* (1913), pp. 50–52.

convicts were not good subjects for discipline and recommended their transferal to the nearby Maryland Hospital for the Insane (on Broadway, at the current site of the Johns Hopkins Hospital). Two years earlier, while visiting the penitentiary, Dorothea Dix saw three convicts whom she described as "decidedly insane . . . but not excited." The plight of the insane, whether inside prison or out, was a life-long concern of Miss Dix,[23] and the visit of this energetic reformer to the penitentiary could have prompted the directors' recommendation. There is no evidence, however, that it was ever carried out on anything like a regular basis. One hindrance was the difficulty in determining those who were truly insane. As noted by the directors in their 1852 *Report,* some convicts feigned insanity to escape labor. Moreover, a lunatic asylum would be understandably reluctant to accept a patient with a criminal history, usually one of violence. The problem of what to do with insane convicts, most of whom could not work or be rehabilitated, would remain for many years.[24]

Another category of criminals requiring special treatment comprised juveniles. For some time prison authorities in Maryland had recognized the pernicious effects of housing very young offenders with older, hardened criminals who could corrupt them. A penitentiary committee recommended in 1828 that youthful offenders be separated from older inmates and confined in separate houses of correction, and the directors in 1830 reported they had classified convicts into "juvenile, adult, and incorrigible" categories and suggested that they be separated and receive different treatment.[25] In 1836 a house of refuge for juvenile offenders was "expected" to be built inside the penitentiary's old west wing, but this was apparently never done, for in 1845 Miss Dix, after describing three such houses she had seen in Boston, New York City, and Philadelphia, noted the absence of a house of refuge for juveniles in Maryland.[26] Her negative observation about Maryland, appearing as it did in an influential pamphlet (two editions in one year), may have helped to keep the project alive: a site was chosen outside the walls of the penitentiary in 1850 and work begun the following year for a reformatory to house white juvenile criminals. It opened in 1855. In

---

[23]*Board of Directors Report* (1876), p. 4, and Marshall, *Dorothea Dix,* pp. 146, 245.

[24]*Board of Directors Report* (1852), p. 7. Over forty years later, Warden John F. Weyler urged the removal of insane convicts to an asylum after their examination by the Lunacy Commission so that they would not be a financial burden to the penitentiary. See *Board of Directors Report* (1889), pp. 9–10. And while visiting the penitentiary in 1987, the present writer was shown a deranged inmate in a locked ward of the prison hospital who had been there for at least ten years.

[25]*Report of Committee Appointed by Board of Directors of Maryland Penitentiary to Visit the Penitentiary and Prisons in the City of Philadelphia and State of New York* (Baltimore: Lucas & Deaver, 1828), p. 25, and *Board of Directors Report* (1830), p. 8.

[26]*Annual Report Boston Prison Discipline Society* (1836), p. 58, and Dix, *Remarks on Prisons and Prison Discipline* (1845), p. 96

the 1869 *Report* Warden John W. Horn protested the confinement of twenty "colored" boys, ages eleven to eighteen, with hardened criminals. Largely at his urging, the House of Refuge and Instruction and Reformation of Colored Children was established in 1872 at Cheltenham, forty-six miles south of Baltimore. Horn served as superintendent for the next ten years before returning to the penitentiary for another stint as warden.[27]

Aside from the special treatment insane convicts and juvenile delinquents clearly required, prison reformers realized they needed to know more about the less obvious differences existing among other inmates in order to give them proper treatment too.[28] As early as 1833, the reformer Francis Lieber had called upon the states (Maryland among them) to provide more accurate and complete statistics about prisoners, including their social background and criminal record, to guide penologists and legislators.[29] Beginning with the Maryland Penitentiary's 1847 *Board of Directors Report,* one finds a marked advance over previous reports with regard to keeping records and organizing statistics, a recognition of their sociological importance. For the first time those officials directly concerned with operating the penitentiary reported separately from the board of directors on the condition and social background of prisoners. In his section, the warden included a cumulative table of punishments (stripes, solitary confinement, cold shower baths) for prisoners of both sexes since 1841; the physician listed those prisoners suffering from various named diseases in a table along with death figures; and the clerk supplied an abstract of prisoners that included notation of their education, drinking habits, and criminal history.

Also, during the 1840s, reformers in the northeastern United States became concerned about the problems of discharged prisoners. Somewhat belatedly, in March 1859, the Relief Association of the Maryland Penitentiary was formed to shield newly discharged convicts from bad influences and to counsel and advise them and help them obtain jobs. The association itself was an offspring of the penitentiary's Sabbath school, established January 1, 1859, to improve morality

---

[27]Wines and Dwight, *Report of the Prisons and Reformatories of the United States and Canada,* p. 399; *Board of Directors Report* (1869), p. 16, and *Biographical Cyclopedia of Representative Men of Maryland and District of Columbia* (Baltimore: National Biographical Company, 1879), p. 412.

[28]David J. Rothman, *The Discovery of the Asylum* (Boston: Little, Brown and Company, 1971), p. 253.

[29]See his introduction to *On the Penitentiary System in the United States and Its Application to France,* by Gustave de Beaumont and Alexis de Tocqueville (1833; repr. New York: Augustus M. Kelley, 1970), pp. xxvii–xxviii. Lieber had a lifelong interest in penology. Beaumont and Tocqueville asked him to translate their book into English, to which he added a thirty-page preface and introduction and copious notes throughout. His views on penology are discussed by Lewis R. Harley in *Francis Lieber: His Life and Political Philosophy* (New York: Columbia University Press, 1899), pp. 137–39. The first known published statistical study of a group of convicts was made in 1832 by the Reverend Jared Curtis, chaplain at the Massachusetts State Penitentiary. See McKelvey, *American Prisons,* p. 20.

One goal of prison reform was to remove children from the presence of hardened inmates. Efforts to do so in Maryland began as early as 1828, but various plans were postponed or dropped until prison reformer Dorothea Dix in 1845 noted the presence of such "houses of refuge" in Boston, New York, and Philadelphia, but not Baltimore. The Baltimore House of Refuge (opposite top), located at the intersection of Frederick Road and Gwynn's Falls, opened in 1855 and soon housed 350 white youths between ten and sixteen years old. "Its object is to save, not punish," noted philanthropist George Brown at the laying of the cornerstone, a sentiment expressed in songs composed for the young population. (From *Hymns and Songs for the Inmates of the Baltimore House of Refuge* [1856]. [Maryland Historical Society.])

HYMNS AND SONGS,
Written for the Inmates of the
HOUSE OF REFUGE, BALTIMORE.

No. 1.
REFUGE HYMN,
Written by Mrs. A. J. G.
SUNG AT THE OPENING OF THE REFUGE.
Spanish Air.
"Go out quickly into the streets and lanes of the city, and bring in hither the poor."—LUKE XIV.

Look from thy dwelling place, Lord and see
This Refuge thy blessing provided;
Here will we gather to train for thee,
The erring, the lost, the misguided.
Wildly they roam
Thro' sins dark way, Lord;
Some without home
Wander astray, Lord;
Save them, we pray!

Here far away
From every snare, Lord;
We'd have them stay
Mercy to share, Lord;
Save them, we pray;

Friends! who have labored with us to raise
This Refuge above us towering,
Let us rejoice and give God the praise,
He bless'd us when all seemed lowering.
Let us go on,
Firm and brave hearted;
Bright breaks the dawn;
Fears have departed;
Hope smiles to-day!
Gather them in,
Lost and neglected;
Tho' marred by sin,
They'll be protected,
Gather them in!

2

No. 2.
PENITENCE.
He which converteth a sinner from the error of his way, shall save a soul from death.—JAMES V.

Tune—"*Thou hast wounded the spirit.*"

From the paths that we ought to have trodden,
We sinfully wandered astray,
And the world hath look'd coldly upon us,
And turn'd us unpitied away;
But friends we have found in this dwelling,
Whose pity and love we have shared,
And our hearts with emotion are swelling,
To know for our souls they have cared.

Then should we not treasure the lessons,
Their kindness has led them to give,
And in penitence turn to the Savior,
Who bids us come to Him and live.
Yes, yes,—we will try to do better,
We know that in Him is our aid,
Though we've sinn'd, yet he'll break every fetter,
On His cross our redemption was paid.

Mrs. A. J. G.

No. 3.
HEBRON.
"God is our refuge and strength, a very present help in trouble."
"The Lord of hosts is with us; the God of Jacob is our refuge."
PSALM—XLVI.

Tune—*Golden Hill.*

Blest be God's holy name,
To Him our thoughts we raise,
O! may His love our hearts inflame,
With hymns of joy and praise.

His mercy who may count!
The universe it fills,
Like Hermon's dew on Zion's mount,
Its living grace distils.

3

A sparrow may not fall,
But at His sov'reign word,
So may the humblest of us all,
Confess Him as our Lord.

The homeless and the poor,
The wayward child of sin,
Neglected, friendless or impure,
All, may His mercy win.

To us His hand is shewn,
We feel His gracious care,
As into paths we have not known,
He leads, His love to share.

Here, all our wants supplied,
We have a Refuge Home,
Lord, to that holier refuge guide,
Where sin no more may come.

O! move each youthful heart,
To listen to thy voice,
To feel the love thou would'st impart,
And in thy rest rejoice.

Sweet rest! that hath no end,
From pain and sorrow free,
Redeemed, our Father and our friend,
To dwell for aye with thee.

J. J. G.

No. 4.
MAGDALEN.
"Come unto me all ye that labor and are heavy laden and I will give you rest."—MATTHEW XI.

Tune—"*Old Folks at home.*"

See, how the forest leaves are fading,
Chill'd by cold dews;
Bright is their many color'd shading,
Brilliant as rainbow hues.
The air is fill'd with stilly gladness,
Yet falls the tear,

10

Slow—full chorus

Refuge dear!
Kindness here
Wipes away our every tear,
Trustingly,
Prayerfully,
To thy care in hope we flee.
Ne'er in sin again to roam,—
Ark of mercy—Refuge home!
God of love,
From above,
Bless our Jubilee!

J. J. G.

NO. 9.
BOYS' EVENING SONG.

Swiss Tune.

Now our daily task is done,
Closely let us gather round,—
Glad and happy, every one
Raise his voice with gleeful sound.
Each to other,
As to brother,
Hand-in-hand, in friendship cling.
Brothers, cheerly—cheerly sing,
Let the chorus loudly ring,
Brothers, cheerly—cheerly sing.

Hark, how echo swells the song!
On the breezy air it floats,
Through the leafy groves along,
Dies away the softened notes.
Oh, the pleasure,
As the measure
On the Summer's breath takes wing.
Hand-in-hand then, cheerly sing,
Let the chorus loudly ring,
Brothers, cheerly—cheerly sing.

11

Lo, the Sun has sunk to rest,
And its rays with ling'ring glow,
Sweetly gild the far-off west;—
Symbol of the love, that now,
Each to other,
As a brother,
Warm and hopeful, here we bring.
Hand-in-hand then, cheerly sing,
Let the chorus loudly ring,
Brothers, cheerly—cheerly sing.

J. J. G.

NO. 10.
CONFESSION.

"Have mercy upon me, O God, according to thy loving kindness; according unto the multitude of thy tender mercies blot out my transgressions—PSALM LI.

Tune—"Morning Light."

Now let our grateful chorus
To thee, ascend, O Lord,
That those who here watch o'er us
Have taught thy Holy word,
By thee the hand was guided
That snatch'd from Satan's snare,
And for our souls provided,
A faithful, saving care.

Lord, grant to us thy blessing,
Thy pardon now bestow,
Humbly our sins confessing,
Before thee, here we bow.
Thou know'st the dark temptation
That led our hearts astray,
Yet free is thy salvation,—
For mercy then we pray.

through Christian religion. Both innovations kindled hope in the prisoners, according to Warden Alfred D. Evans, who concluded his report in 1859 on an enlightened note: "Thus I find a moral control over my charge is stronger than the lash."[30]

Other concerns at this time for the well-being of prisoners were not wanting either. A tobacco allowance had been initiated as early as 1845.[31] Then in 1848 the board of directors acknowledged the donation of 350 books to form the nucleus of a prison library. In 1852 the warden asked that lighting be available in the dungeon-like cells for those men who wanted to read during the long winter evenings, and five years later the newly established prison library of a thousand volumes proved useful to those prisoners idled by the fire that destroyed the north wing workshop. Much later, in his report for 1883, Warden John W. Horn noted a large addition to the prison library, bringing it up to about two thousand volumes, but added that "sensational and pernicious books and papers" were excluded.[32]

In addressing themselves to the multifaceted problem of reforming those placed in their care, prison officials in Maryland did not work in isolation. To learn how other prisons were being run, they turned to the annual reports of the Boston Prison Discipline Society, which from 1826 until 1854 served as the most important source for information about prison administrations throughout the country. The directors of the Maryland Penitentiary consulted these reports regularly, as seen for example in their own annual report for 1851. Here they not only showed their familiarity with the financial performances of other prisons in the eastern United States but when discussing the Western Penitentiary of Pennsylvania and State Prison of New Jersey used the same language and figures provided by the Boston Prison Discipline Society report the previous year.[33]

The Boston Prison Discipline Society had been founded and organized in 1825 by the Reverend Louis Dwight, an ardent promoter of the Auburn penal system (congregate work during the day in silence) and a man who believed in providing bibles, Sunday schools, and resident chaplains for prisoners. Dwight had already left his mark on the Maryland Penitentiary physically. He had helped design the five-tier eastern dormitory (1829) by giving it an arcade interior—a

---

[30]McKelvey, *American Prisons*, pp. 42, 59; *First Annual Report of the Relief Association of the Maryland Penitentiary* (1860), pp. 5–6, and the *Board of Directors Report* (1859), pp. 22–23. The earlier introduction of Sunday schools by the Society of Friends for male and female prisoners is noted in the *Board of Directors Report* (1846), pp. 12–13, but this experiment was apparently short-lived.

[31]*Board of Directors Report* (1847), p. 12.

[32]*Board of Directors Report* (1848), p. 6; (1852), p. 14; (1857), p. 12; and (1883), p. 4.

[33]McKelvey, *American Prisons*, p. 20; *Board of Directors Report* (1851), pp. 9–11.

central open space from floor to ceiling—that allowed observation of all cell doors by one person. This same feature also allowed a preacher to stand between the cells so that all could hear his voice on Sunday morning. A bible was placed in each cell, but prison officials failed to provide a strong Sunday school program or resident chaplain, both of which Dwight thought necessary for the reformation of the convicts.[34] The 1837 report of the Boston Prison Discipline Society noted that religious services at the Maryland Penitentiary were volunteered by different clergy in Baltimore, and a Sunday school continued for several years only through the efforts of voluntary superintendents and teachers.[35] Like many volunteer programs, this one waned, for in 1846 another Sunday school was established at the penitentiary by the Society of Friends, and still another in 1859. And later, in his report for 1866, the warden expressed his belief that the Maryland Penitentiary was the only institution in the country without a permanently attached chaplain. Clergymen were still being "invited" to preach at the penitentiary in 1878.[36]

Despite failing to provide a strong religious program, the Maryland Penitentiary took part in the development of a reform movement in the 1860s from the very outset. When the newly organized American Association for the Improvement of Prison Discipline convened in 1860, Maryland was one of eight states to send its representatives. After being interrupted by the Civil War, the movement resumed under the leadership of Enoch C. Wines, who with Theodore Dwight published the landmark *Report of the Prisons and Reformatories of the United States and Canada* in 1867, which, as noted above, seems to have directly influenced the reform-minded warden, John W. Horn. Wines went on to found the National Prison Association, which held its second meeting in Baltimore in 1873. This meeting was attended by the influential G. S. Griffith, president of the Maryland Prisoners' Aid Society, and from the penitentiary by Warden Thomas S. Wilkinson, Director Henry Seim, and Clerk R. V. Page. At the conclusion of the meeting, the members of the National Prison Association voted their thanks to the Maryland Prisoners' Aid Society for having made all the preparations.[37]

The greatest threat to the reformation of prisoners during this period came from overcrowding. As the city grew, so of course did its prison population, especially during times of economic depression such as the panic of 1857. In

---

[34]McKelvey, *American Prisons*, pp. 15, 20, 37; *Board of Directors Report* (1828), p. 10; Crawford, *Report on the Penitentiaries of the United States* (1835), p. 95.

[35]*Boston Prison Discipline Society* (1837), p. 56.

[36]*Board of Directors Report* (1847), pp. 12–13; (1859), p. 22; (1866), p. 12; and (1878), p. 12.

[37]McKelvey, *American Prisons*, pp. 65, 66–68, 70, 74–75, 88–89. *Transactions of the National Prison Reform Congress: Held at Baltimore, Maryland, January 21–24, 1873, Being the Second Annual Meeting of the National Prison Association of the United States* (Baltimore, 1873), pp. 319, 481.

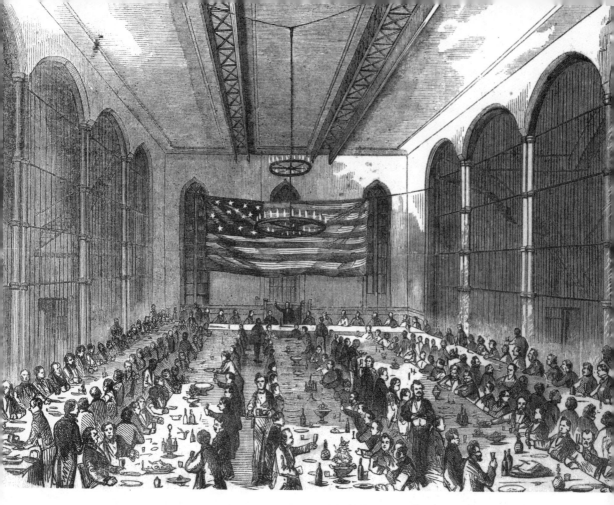

In 1859, the rapidly growing city of Baltimore built a new City Jail on the same location. This engraving of the grand ceremonial banquet marking the occasion appeared in *Frank Leslie's Illustrated Newspaper*. (Maryland Historical Society.)

that year the warden reported a shortage of single cells—only 256 for an average population of 413—forcing him to lodge seven and eight prisoners together in some rooms. Inasmuch as construction had already begun on the new City Jail adjacent to the west wall of the penitentiary, he urged the purchase of ground to expand the penitentiary northward. Dr. Charles Frick, perhaps the most distinguished physician ever to serve at the penitentiary, also deplored the overcrowding, blaming it for the increase in sickness and mortality of the prisoners. Not only were six or seven of them to be found in one room, he said, but "oftentimes two and three in [the] same bed, in utter violation of the law. That anything like moral reformation can take place is out of the question; . . . that proper discipline of the prison can be preserved under these circumstances is simply ridiculous." Conditions in the male hospital were worse, he said, forty crowded in a room sixty by forty feet, "all so closely packed, that I have with difficulty made

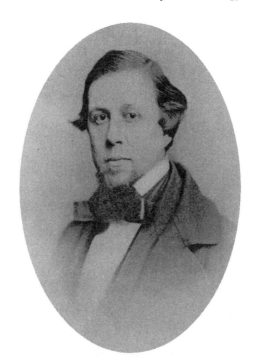

Dr. Charles Frick, 1823–1860. (From Cordell's *Medical Annals of Maryland.*)

my way to the sick man's bedside, when summoned to his assistance, in the night. In an atmosphere poisoned as this is, I hesitate to perform the most trivial surgical operation, and look with anxiety on any case of injury admitted involving a wound of the flesh." In 1859 the directors again urged the purchase of the vacant land to the north for expansion and Warden Alfred D. Evans, noting the dilapidation of the older buildings, cried, "For the honor of the state, give us a new prison."[38]

Just prior to this appeal occurred two events which in retrospect seem like omens of the war that would worsen the overcrowding, postpone new dormitory construction, and in various other ways hinder the reformation of the penitentiary's prisoners. On October 24, 1855, "Negro Bob" Butler, a former slave and the penitentiary's first prisoner, died at age sixty-six of "softening of the brain." He had served forty-four years there and at his own request was buried in the prison yard.[39]

The second event was played up in the northern newspapers as part of the

---

[38] *Board of Directors Report* (1857), pp. 3, 9–10, 32–34; and (1859), pp. 16, 20. Charles Frick came to the penitentiary in 1849 and served until 1857. His annual reports on the health of the prisoners far surpassed those of his predecessors in both comprehensiveness and detail. His short but illustrious career as a physician, scholar, and teacher is summarized by Dr. John R. Quinan in *Medical Annals of Baltimore from 1608 to 1880* (Baltimore: Press of Isaac Friedenwald, 1884), pp. 100–101.

[39]"Sketch of the Maryland Penitentiary," *Board of Directors Report* (1881), p. 41.

gathering storm that led to the Civil War. Samuel Green, born about 1802, a free black from Dorchester County, was sentenced in 1857 to ten years in the Maryland Penitentiary for having in his possession a copy of *Uncle Tom's Cabin*. This book, along with a map of Canada and a railroad schedule to that country also found in his possession, were regarded as "inflammatory abolition materials designed to create discontent and insurrectionary tendencies in blacks" and found to violate legislation passed in 1831 and 1841 in reaction to the Nat Turner revolt. While Green was quietly serving his time, the affair became a *cause célèbre* in the North and an embarrassment to the South.[40]

As the sectional conflict worsened in 1860, Maryland—a border state with strong commercial ties to both the North and South—experienced a crisis of conflicting loyalties. When war broke out in April 1861, it appeared that parts of the state, especially southern Maryland and the city of Baltimore, had enough strength to wrench it out of the Union. But the issue did not remain in doubt for long. On May 14, 1861, General Benjamin F. Butler placed his Union cannon on Federal Hill overlooking Baltimore, and by autumn the presence of Federal troops at other strategic locations in the city and throughout the state had secured Maryland for the Union. Though spared the physical shock of the battles to come, the penitentiary would feel the effects of the war indirectly.

Even before the first shots were fired the penitentiary suffered financially. In 1860 the uncertainty of Maryland's commitment to the North or to the South sent the state's economy into a depression, which, augmented by the ensuing war, would last two years. Beginning in 1861 a Federal blockade of the southern states stopped the flow of raw materials and the sale of finished products for two of the prison's industries. "Great difficulty has been found in employing the prisoners," the penitentiary board of directors stated in 1862, "owing to the stagnation of business of almost every kind, arising from the peculiar state of the country."[41] Unemployed prisoners were, of course, that much less amenable to discipline.

Less verifiable was the effect the war might have had on the attitude of the prisoners toward the penal institution designed to reform them. The number of rebellious incidents reported at this time—the first in over a quarter of a cen-

---

[40]He would be released five years later midway through his sentence after being pardoned by Governor Augustus Williamson Bradford on condition that he leave the state within sixty days. See Richard Albert Blondo, "Samuel Green: A Black Life in Antebellum Maryland" (M.A. thesis, University of Maryland, 1988), pp. 25, 29, 63–66.

[41]Richard Walsh and William Lloyd Fox, *Maryland: A History* (Annapolis: Hall of Records Commission, Dept. of General Services, 1983), pp. 333–34, 346; *Report and Accompanying Documents of the House Committee Appointed to Examine into the Affairs of the Maryland Penitentiary* (Frederick, Md.: B. H. Richardson, Printer, 1861), pp. 4–6; "Sketch of the Maryland Penitentiary," *Board of Directors Report* (1881), p. 78.

tury—suggests that discord in the world outside the prison walls also made the convicts less tractable. On a Sunday afternoon, two days before Christmas, 1860, four black convicts set fire with a slow match to a brick cooper shop, causing an estimated loss of $30,000 and destroying the contractor's business there.[42] On a Friday afternoon, June 7, 1861, black convict John Brown, wielding a razor, severely cut Deputy Warden Isaac G. Roberts just as Roberts was about to punish him for "impudent conduct." Brown was shot in the ensuing scuffle and died of his wounds several days later.[43] On a Saturday morning, July 26, 1862, convict William Lynch, while painting the two small guardhouses at the front gate, used a rope to escape over the wall. And on August 8 of the same year, Andrew J. Hoff, confined to a dark punishment cell for assaulting a fellow prisoner, dug his way with an iron bucket hoop into an adjoining cell that was vacant and unlocked. He hid until dark and then escaped over the wall. Neither prisoner was ever recaptured, despite liberal rewards.[44]

More incidents like these were reported in the ensuing twenty or so years than ever before in the penitentiary's long history. Three convicts escaped in 1866. On January 17, 1875, during Sunday dinner, black convict Justin Shipley tried to brain a guard with an iron bar, was shot three times, and caused a near riot among the six hundred prisoners. Next year, on August 25, black convict John Thomas assaulted an armless civilian foreman in the marble shop with a knife and then cut the foreman's brother who had come to his rescue. There were suicides, too. That same year convict William Relt hanged himself in his cell. Another suicide by hanging was reported two years later, as well as the death of a convict after having cut his own throat several months earlier. On March 1, 1882, convict Robert Taylor was shot and killed in the foundry by a deputy keeper for being insubordinate. And next year, on January 6, convict Rupert Spencer jumped from an upper tier to the basement and died in the hospital.[45]

As one might expect, the end of the war increased the problem of overcrowding at the penitentiary. Not all the demobilized soldiers and freed slaves could find employment, and some of these turned to petty crime. In 1865, the year hostilities ceased, the directors reported among the new prisoners received "an extraordinary number of colored women, boys and men for short terms [i.e.

---

[42] *Report and Accompanying Documents of the House Committee Appointed to Examine into the Affairs of the Maryland Penitentiary* (Frederick, Md.: B. H. Richardson, Printer, 1861), pp. 10–11, 35. One of the arsonists was named Samuel Green, the same as the abolitionist described above, but there is no evidence they were the same person.

[43] *Baltimore Sun,* June 12, 1861.

[44] *Baltimore Sun,* July 29, 1862; *Board of Directors Report* (1862), p. 10.

[45] *Board of Directors Report* (1866), p. 7; *Baltimore Sun,* January 19, 1875 and August 26, 1876; *Board of Directors Report* (1876), p. 10; *Board of Directors Report* (1878), p. 10, 33; *Board of Directors Report* (1883), p. 12.

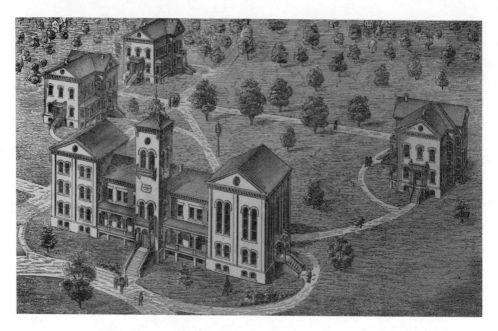

Built at the urging of penitentiary warden John W. Horn in response to postwar overcrowding and harsh conditions in the prison, the House of Reformation for Colored Children opened in 1872 at Cheltenham, forty-six miles south of Baltimore. In his 1869 *Report,* Warden Horn protested the confinement of twenty "colored" boys, ages eleven to eighteen, with hardened criminals. (Maryland Historical Society.)

six months or less}."[46] Two years later the directors reported an "astonishing" number of new prisoners received, the number of blacks quadrupling—only the governor's clemency (use of his pardoning power) prevented disastrous over-crowding.[47] They renewed their appeal for the expansion of the penitentiary northward. By 1869 the penitentiary population had reached an all-time high of 687, of whom 179 (or one quarter) were between the ages of twelve and twenty. This included yet another increase in black prisoners, who the directors said came mostly from the counties and, being used to agriculture, had diffi-culty in learning mechanical skills. The directors made a long and eloquent plea for more dormitory space, claiming that it was impossible to herd sixty or more prisoners into a room built for twenty. The penitentiary physician called condi-tions "repulsive . . . discreditable" and blamed the overcrowding for the large number of blacks dying of consumption.[48]

---

[46]*Board of Directors Report* (1865), p. 6. A year later, the directors attributed this great increase in black prisoners to the fact that formerly their masters punished them for petty crimes; now, as free men, they were sentenced by the court to the penitentiary (*Board of Directors Report,* 1866, p. 9). The House of Correction would not be open for petty offenders until 1878.

[47]*Board of Directors Report* (1867), pp. 5, 8.

[48]*Board of Directors Report* (1869), pp. 5, 8–9, 12, 38–42.

These appeals at last were heeded. The legislature opened its pursestrings, not enough for the requested expansion northward with the planned construction of a modern prison complex, but enough for the penitentiary to meet its growing needs piecemeal by improving existing buildings and constructing additional dormitory space within its old boundaries. The major improvements were as follows. In 1870 an entirely new brick dormitory building five stories high and measuring 100 by 25 feet was built to house 160 female prisoners,[49] as was an adjoining three-story matron's residence (60 by 18 feet) with rooms for a female chapel and Sabbath school. The two-story brick building (110 by 50 feet)[50] that housed the men's dining room (lower floor) and a dormitory (upper floor) was raised two stories to provide space for religious services, and a workshop or dormitory, according to need. One of the old congregate dormitories was gutted and raised to six stories, then 344 single cells built into its outer walls, each having independent ventilation.[51] All of these improvements, the directors noted, were done by the prisoners themselves, who even forged the doors and bars and locks for the cells, thus saving the state much money.[52]

In 1876 another female dormitory was added, and a year later the arrival of federal prisoners resulted in a five-story building (97 by 25 feet) being erected for 100 males called "Central Dormitory." Yet another five-story male dormitory (102 by 43 feet) was built in 1878, when the prison population reached a temporary peak of 984. Thereafter it decreased sharply, falling to 534 by 1881. Two reasons were offered for this great decline: a general improvement in the economy ("better the times, better the people") and the recent completion of the House of Correction (1878), which now took in the petty offenders who would otherwise have been sent to the penitentiary.[53] This build-up of the penitentiary from 1870 through 1878 had not only relieved the conditions of overcrowding but actually left the institution with an overcapacity that lasted until its final expansion northward in the 1890s, with the construction of the granite buildings still standing at the corner of Eager and Forrest streets.

As the 1870s ended, the penitentiary found itself in better financial condition than ever before in its seventy-year history. It had just completed its most prosperous decade since the 1820s, owing to a better postwar economy, but

---

[49]Later designated C dormitory, this brick building was encased in a granite shell in 1906–7 and later equipped with 135 steel cells for housing female prisoners. See *Board of Directors Report* (1906), pp. 14–15. It is still in use, housing male prisoners.

[50]Formerly the east wing of the radial workshop complex built in 1836, this building with its two additional stories still survives and is known as the State Use or G building.

[51]I have been unable to trace this building in the older maps.

[52]*Board of Directors Report* (1871), pp. 4, 6–7.

[53]"A Sketch of the Maryland Penitentiary," *Board of Directors Report* (1881), pp. 82–86.

Overleaf: The City Jail and penitentiary appear in the upper right of this photograph, taken in 1873 from a church steeple. (Maryland Historical Society.)

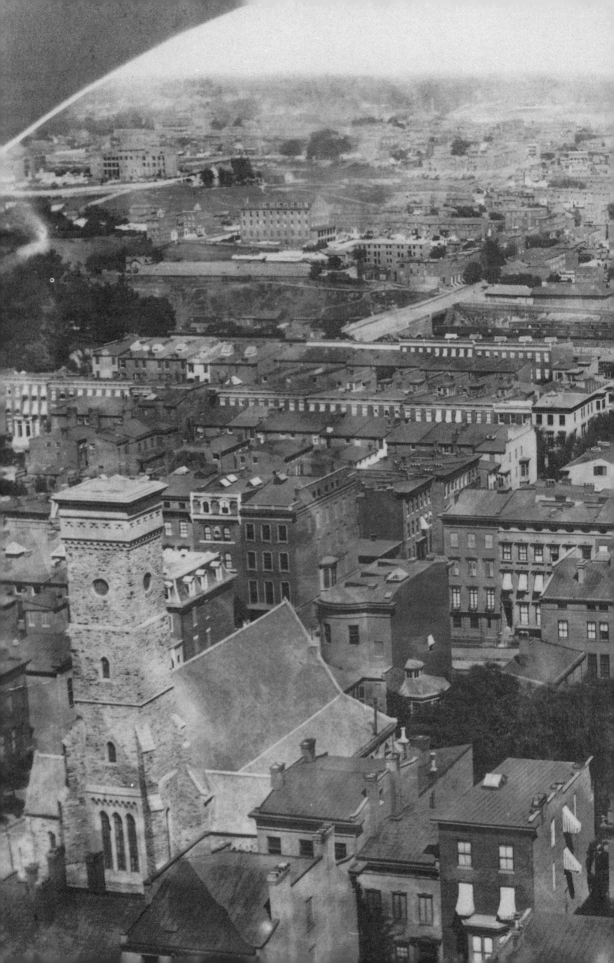

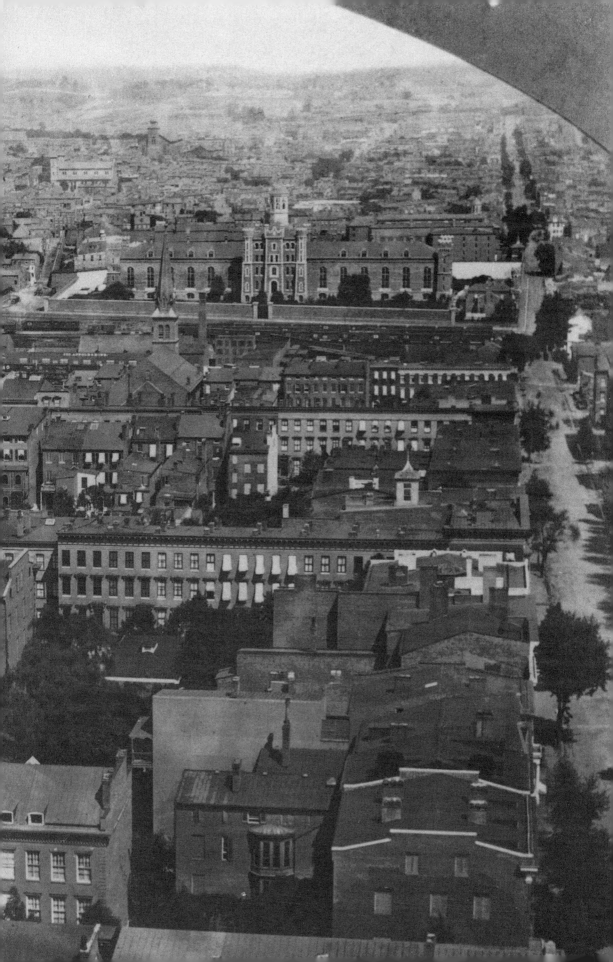

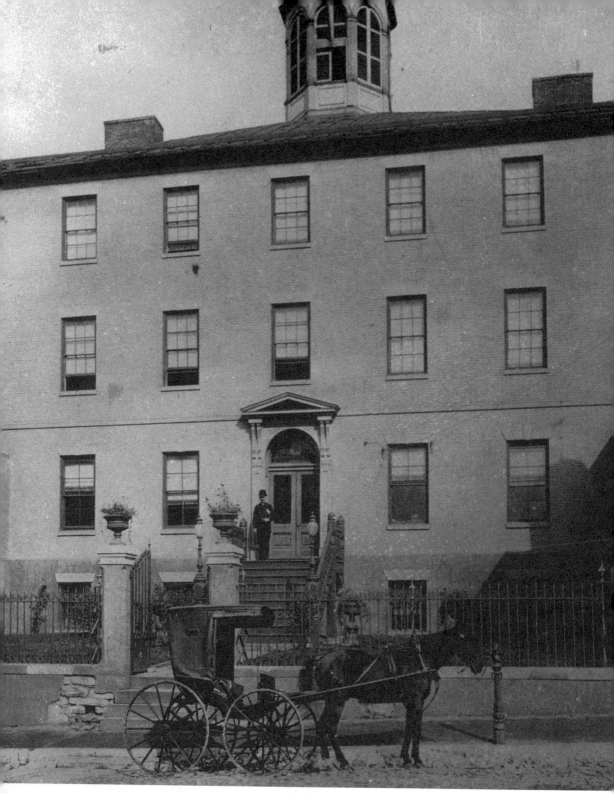

This earliest known surviving photograph of the penitentiary's original administration building was probably taken in the mid-1880s when Warden John W. Horn (wearing the derby hat) was serving his second tour of duty (May 4, 1882–May 30, 1888). (Courtesy, Lt. James Felix.)

John W. Horn, a regimental commander of Maryland Union volunteers during the Civil War, was the most progressive, reform-minded warden at the Maryland penitentiary in the nineteenth century. Convicts were "still human beings capable of being made better, and not to be treated as brutes because of their moral bankruptcy," he wrote. Horn served two terms, 1867–72 and 1882–88. (From *Biographical Encyclopedia of Representative Men of Maryland and the District of Columbia* [Baltimore: National Biographical Publishing Company, 1879].)

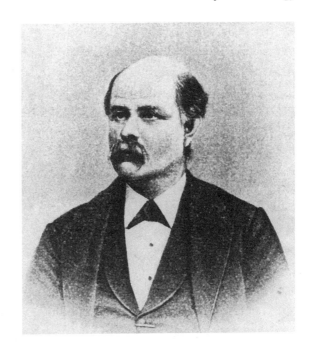

especially to the more widespread use of the contract labor system at the penitentiary. For the time being, at least, it had achieved one of its main goals: to become self-supporting.[54] Its other main goal—the reformation of prisoners—proved more elusive because of penology's many facets.

The prison had responded well to most of the new theories or ideas in penology advanced during this period. Brutal discipline had been mitigated, if not eliminated; a commutation ("good time") law had been carried out by 1876; and improved record-keeping, especially of convicts' social backgrounds, led to recognition of the differences between the insane, juvenile delinquents, and petty offenders. Although the proper disposition of insane convicts would remain a problem, the recognition of the special needs of juvenile and petty offenders led to a rudimentary system of classification and the building of reformatories (1855, 1873) and a house of correction (1878). The needs of discharged prisoners were recognized by the establishment of the Relief Association of the Maryland Penitentiary in 1859.

In 1879, Enoch C. Wines, father of the reform era that had just ended, praised the penitentiary. He pronounced the institution "one of the best managed and most successful in the country both morally and financially." Still, he went on to say, "there is a grave defect which so excellent an establishment ought to supply without unnecessary delay; that is, the want of a prison school and schoolmaster.

---

[54]Ibid., pp. 80, 82, 85.

It is a neglect which amounts to a reproach, an injustice, when the prisoners pay all the bills and return a surplus into the State treasury."[55]

As the 1880s began, the penitentiary directors promised they would strive "to perpetuate the successful era which has existed for nearly ten years past, and feel confident of accomplishing their purpose."[56] In 1882 the reform-minded John W. Horn returned to the penitentiary for his second tour of duty as warden and for the next four years presided over the continuing sound financial health of the institution. But at the end of 1887 the penitentiary was left with the very small surplus of $661.76, which the directors attributed primarily to the Davis Shoe Company's withdrawal from its contract, an action that threw a large number of prisoners out of work. The board also reported mounting anti-prison labor sentiment by "mechanics" throughout the country and the enactment of anti-prison labor laws by different states. Warden Horn added that one-half of those prisoners not on contract were non-productive "by reason of old age, loss of limb, or other physical infirmity. . . . These wrecks of humanity . . . commit petty larcenies for which they are sent to prison, to be fed and warmed at the expense of the State, and consume what is earned by the labor of others. The Jails and Almhouses are always full of them, like the ebb and flow of the sea they come and go, out in the morning and back at night and in the end find their way here."[57] But while mindful of the need for the penitentiary to support itself financially, Warden Horn believed that convicts were "still human beings capable of being made better, and not to be treated as brutes because of their moral bankruptcy, or their blood coined into money to enrich individuals [i.e., contractors], or the State saved from any financial responsibility in the management of its prisoners."[58]

While the building program from 1870 through 1878 had temporarily relieved the problem of overcrowding, the penitentiary at the close of the 1880s remained an outmoded prison, a patchwork of brick buildings with dungeon-like cells lacking proper ventilation, heat, light, and plumbing. During his last year as warden (1887), Horn worked the prisoners hard at repairs and improvements and pronounced the prison "in better condition now than at any other time in its history." But, he went on to say, "no amount of time, labor or money can ever modernize it, or make it creditable to the State. The lot is far from being large enough, less than five acres, most of the buildings are old and some

---

[55] *The State of Prisons and of Child-Saving Institutions in the United States* (1880; repr. Montclair, N.J.: Patterson Smith, 1968), p. 211.

[56] "A Sketch of the Maryland Penitentiary," *Board of Directors Report* (1881), p. 68.

[57] *Board of Directors Report* (1887), pp. 3, 6.

[58] Ibid., p. 10.

of them badly ventilated, and all the sleeping cells too small." He called for steam heat and electric lights to replace the "dangerous and unsavory coal oil lamps," which would allow the prisoners more opportunity "for improving their minds by the reading of good books, during the long hours of winter, from dark to nine p.m."[59]

The expansion of the prison northward and the construction of a modern prison with steel cellblocks, plumbing, steam heat and electric lights would take more money than the state had ever appropriated at one time for the Maryland Penitentiary. The realization of Warden Horn's vision would not take place until after his retirement and the earnest efforts of his successor, John F. Weyler.

---

[59]Ibid., p. 9.

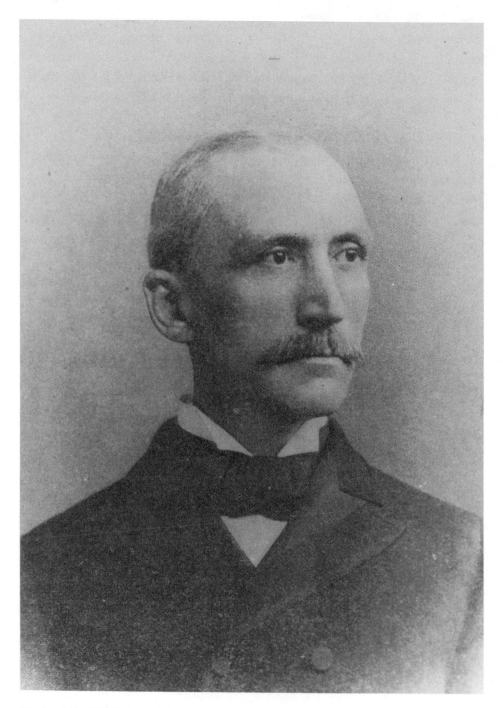

Warden John F. Weyler ruled the penitentiary from 1888 to 1912, earning widespread praise for making the institution profitable, but investigations proved his administration both cruel and corrupt. He is shown here in 1899, at the height of his power. (From the 1899 *Annual Report of the Board of Directors of the Maryland Penitentiary.*)

Chapter Four

The Rise and Fall of Warden John F. Weyler

1888 – 1920

"This is a walled kingdom and you know who the king is."
—Sidney Johnson, "colored" convict, testifying before the
Maryland Penitentiary Penal Commission in 1912[1]

On May 31, 1888, the president of the Baltimore City Council, John F. Weyler, was sworn in as warden of the Maryland Penitentiary.[2] He ruled there for the next twenty-four years, longer than any predecessor. During his long tenure he pushed through the construction of the massive granite penitentiary at the corner of Eager and Forrest streets in Baltimore and turned its annual operating deficits into surpluses—all the while acquiring power and prestige until at his retirement in 1912 a grateful General Assembly awarded him the specially created title of warden emeritus and a lucrative sinecure at the penitentiary. His reputation as a "model" warden was abruptly shattered less than a year later upon publication of the *Report of Maryland Penitentiary Penal Commission* (1913), charging his administration with mismanagement, cruelty, and corruption. It is a story with tragic overtones, about a man who guided the penitentiary through a crucial period in its evolution from a haphazard accumulation of nineteenth-century brick buildings into a planned

---

[1] The Maryland Penitentiary Penal Commission, Stenographic Record of Testimony (1912), 1:285, Maryland Room, Enoch Pratt Free Library. Hereafter cited as Penal Commission Testimony.
[2] *Baltimore Sun,* June 1, 1888.

modern prison with steel cellblocks and who operated it with machine-like efficiency. Ironically, this very efficiency, apparently achieved through harsh disciplinary methods and without regard to the rehabilitation of the convicts, ultimately led to his downfall.

Born on February 8, 1844,[3] Weyler was listed in the 1873 Baltimore City directory as a saloon keeper with a residence at 25 Brown Street, which ran along the south side of the Cross Street market in Baltimore's Seventeenth Ward.[4] Undoubtedly the nature of his work eased his entry into the political life of this working-class community, and by 1876 he had achieved a position of considerable importance—he issued licenses for stalls as clerk of the Cross Street Market.[5]

His rise in the larger political world of Baltimore City came about through his early involvement in the Democratic Party machine, whose boss, Isaac Freeman Rasin, ruled the city from the 1870s to 1895.[6] Rasin controlled the city council and picked its nominees from each ward. In October 1879, Weyler was elected to the second branch of the council from the Seventeenth Ward.[7] Unbeatable thereafter, he served on all the important standing committees, steadily gaining experience and political influence until in 1888 his colleagues named him city council president.[8] Early that same year, as he began his term, he was appointed warden of the Maryland Penitentiary by Rasin's close ally, state party boss and U.S. Senator Arthur Pue Gorman.[9]

---

[3]According to the *Baltimore American,* February 9, 1913, Weyler celebrated his sixty-ninth birthday on the previous day. However, the 1880 census, taken June 8, listed him as being aged thirty-nine, that is, born in 1841. This appears to have been a clerical error.

[4]His background was not only humble but somewhat obscure. A search of the sacramental books of churches in the vicinity has turned up no record of his baptism or of his marriage to his wife, Louisa (listed in the 1880 census as being aged thirty-three). Having been born in 1841 or 1844, Weyler could have served in the Civil War but is not listed in Daniel Hartzler's comprehensive *Marylanders in the Confederacy* (Silver Spring, Md.: Family Line Publications, 1986) or in L. Allison Wilmer, et al., *History of the Maryland Volunteers Civil War* (Baltimore: Guggenheimer, Weil & Co., 1899).

[5]WPA File, 1876 document #2406, "Market Stall," Baltimore City Archives. On May 1, 1879, Weyler issued a license slip (document #524-C) to his wife, Louisa, for a permanent stall, presumably—with his growing political importance—in a good location inside the market house, not outside under the eaves.

[6]In 1912 Frank Furst, president of the board of penitentiary directors, told the Maryland Penitentiary Penal Commission that he had first known Weyler forty years previously, when the Democratic Party was being formed in Baltimore City (Penal Commission Testimony, 1:205). The formation of the Democratic machine in Baltimore and rise of Rasin are described by James B. Crooks in *Politics & Progress: The Rise of Urban Progressivism in Baltimore 1895–1911* (Baton Rouge: Louisiana State University Press, 1968), pp. 6–13.

[7]WPA File, document #159, "Judges of Election," Baltimore City Archives. According to former city archivist Tom Hollowak, second branch members of the council were junior to those designated first branch. The distinction between the two branches was somewhat vague, being originally based on property qualifications, but in any case by Weyler's time a member could move easily from one branch to the other.

[8]"Officers of the Corporation" (1888), p. 6. At the time, city council presidents were elected not by the public but by the other members of the council.

[9]For Weyler's appointment by Senator Gorman, see Frank Furst in Penal Commission Testimony, 1:205. On the alliance of Rasin and Gorman, see Crooks, *Politics & Progress,* p. 11, and John R. Lambert in *Arthur Pue Gorman* (Baton Rouge: Louisiana State University Press, 1953), pp. 31–37.

The appointment came as a surprise, and not just because of its timing. Completely innocent of prison experience, Weyler entered upon his duties, he admitted, "with some misgivings."[10] His long-time friend Frank Furst later recalled, "I thought it was a mistake and Weyler thought it was a mistake."[11] But it seems unlikely that Senator Gorman would have risked his own or his party's reputation by making a careless choice. As a successful party boss and shrewd judge of men, he must have recognized his appointee's administrative talent. Weyler's work in the Democratic Party had already earned him the reputation of being "a thoroughly practical politician,"[12] that is, one who knew how to keep the party machinery running smoothly. His rise in the city council hierarchy had also shown executive ability and leadership qualities. A forceful administrator was needed to replace the retiring warden, Gen. John W. Horn.[13] After the swearing-in ceremony on May 31, 1888, Weyler received no indoctrination from Horn other than a five-minute talk and a brief tour of the penitentiary. What Weyler saw was discouraging: "The buildings were a wreck and the discipline poor. Conditions were in a chaotic state."[14]

He did not exaggerate by much, if at all. Physically the penitentiary was essentially the same as pictured in the Sachse *Bird's Eye View* of 1869. It occupied a four-acre site adjacent to the City Jail, bounded by Truxton Street to the north, Forrest to the east, and Madison to the south. Within its twenty-foot-high walls lay a collection of brick buildings that had accumulated at random since the early nineteenth century.[15] In the upper yard, above the inner bisecting wall, were the workshops completed in 1836. In the lower yard, below the bisecting wall and fronting Madison, were the three original buildings: a square, three-story administration building (1811) flanked by two narrow wings, G dormitory (1829) to the east and B dormitory (1811) to the west, with a fourth building, C dormitory, added alongside the west wing in 1870.[16] The dormitory cells were small (three

---

[10]Annual Report of the Warden, 1888, p. 2, Maryland State Archives.

[11]Penal Commission Testimony, 1:205.

[12]Frank R. Kent, *The Story of Maryland Politics* (Baltimore: Thomas and Evans Co., 1911), pp. 77, 117.

[13]John Watt Horn (1834–97) served in the Union army and for a total of eleven years was warden of the Maryland Penitentiary (from May 16, 1867 to May 15, 1872 and from May 4, 1882 to May 30, 1888). See *The Biographical Cyclopedia of Representative Men of Maryland and District of Columbia* (Baltimore: National Biographical Co., 1879), pp. 411–12.

[14]*Baltimore Sun*, May 2, 1912.

[15]John H. B. Latrobe, *Picture of Baltimore* (Baltimore: F. Lucas, 1832), p. 86, and J. C. Myers, *Sketches on a Tour through the Northern and Eastern States, the Canadas & Nova Scotia* (Harrisonburg, Va.: J. H. Wartmann & Bros., 1849), p. 35.

[16]Both the sixty-foot-square administration building and its adjoining west wing (B dormitory) were completed and ready to receive the first convicts in 1811. See Thomas W. Griffith, *Annals of Baltimore* (Baltimore: William Woody, 1824), pp. 197–98. The east wing (G dormitory) was completed in 1829, the workshops in 1836. See *Testimony Taken Before the Joint Commission of the Legislature on the Penitentiary* (Annapolis, 1837), pp. 9, 12. The fourth building, C dormitory, was added alongside the west wing in 1870. See J. Thomas Scharf, *History of Baltimore City and County* (1881, repr. Baltimore: Regional Publishing Co., 1971), p. 203.

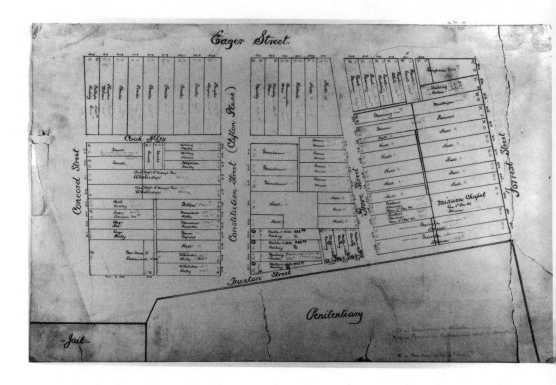

Above: An 1894 plat map, just before the penitentiary began its expansion northward from the old yard. (Maryland State Archives.)
Below: Original drawing of the new penitentiary by architect Jackson C. Gott, showing the south wing extended all the way to Madison Street. The south wing was never completed for lack of funds. (Maryland State Archives.)

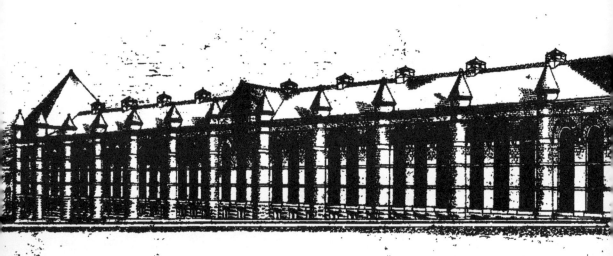

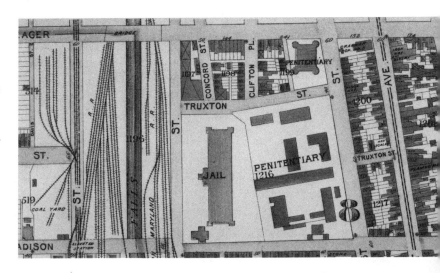

Right: The *Bromley Atlas of Baltimore,* 1896, shows the new administration building at the corner of Eager and Forrest Streets. The west and south wings would come later. *Below right:* Gott's drawing for the planned expansion.(Maryland State Archives.)

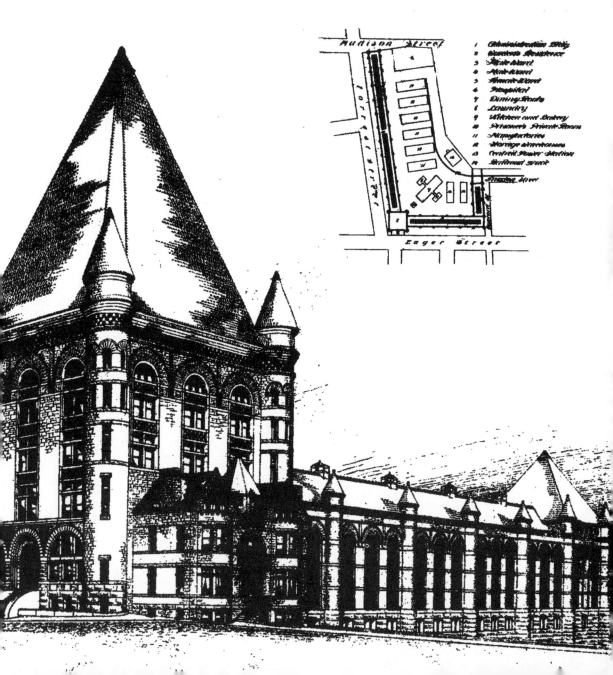

and one-half feet wide by nine feet long by seven feet high) and dungeon-like (some without windows and others with only four-inch slits, secured with iron-slatted doors, having no wash bowls or toilets and furnished only with "filth buckets."[17]

Poor discipline adversely affected the penitentiary's financial health, which was already in a precarious condition. The institution was supposed to support itself by contract labor, a program still in wide use at penitentiaries throughout the nation but gradually being phased out because of labor-union opposition.[18] Under this system the state leased convict labor to private manufacturers, who then assigned prisoners a daily "task" or quota in the penitentiary shops. The system also was supposed to give convicts a chance to earn some money for themselves by exceeding the daily quota ("overtask"). Failure to reach the daily quota, either through convicts' laziness or rebelliousness (acts of sabotage were not uncommon) meant the penitentiary operated at a loss.[19] The Davis Shoe Company recently had broken off its contract with the prison.[20]

Weyler took immediate steps to improve productivity by bringing in a new contractor, the Baltimore Boot and Shoe Company, and tightening discipline. He had prison rules revised and reprinted "so that now," he reported, "we are working under a perfect system which is rigidly enforced." He discouraged malingerers by requiring shopworkers to sign up for sick call ahead of time.[21] Prisoners who refused to work were whipped with the "cat" (cat-o'-nine-tails), as was still the practice at some other prisons in the country.[22]

Meanwhile, the antiquated facilities cried out for attention. In his first full year Weyler had inmates renovate and repaint the dormitories and shops. Now, he reported, "these old buildings present a creditable appearance." A new dining room and kitchen boiler made it possible to give all convicts an early breakfast, adding more time for work. Special quarters were fitted up in C dormitory for the insane, to give them "cheerful and healthy" surroundings. He renewed the plea, also made by his predecessor, for steam heat and electric lighting. He urged the renewal of the "fearfully dilapidated" boardwalks on top of the walls

---

[17] *Annual Report of the Board of Directors* (1913), p. 10. Hereafter *Board of Directors Report.*

[18] Blake McKelvey, *American Prisons: A History of Good Intentions* (Montclair, N.J.: Patterson Smith, 1977), pp. 250–51.

[19] The contract labor system was introduced at the Maryland Penitentiary in the mid-nineteenth century but did not earn enough for the institution to become fully self-supporting until the third year of Weyler's administration. See *Report of the Maryland Penitentiary Penal Commission* (Baltimore: State of Maryland, 1913), Appendix B, p. 311. Hereafter *Penal Commission Report.*

[20] *Board of Directors Report* (1887), p. 3.

[21] *Board of Directors Report* (1889), pp. 11–12, 30–31.

[22] McKelvey, *American Prisons*, p. 189. In nearby Delaware, flogging persisted longer than in any other state, over 1,600 whippings being administered between 1900 and 1945. See Robert Caldwell, *Red Hannah: Delaware's Whipping Post* (Philadelphia: University of Pennsylvania Press, 1947), p. 1.

and the paving of prison roadbeds and muddy yards with Belgian blocks "on account of their durability and cleanliness."[23]

But much more was needed, as Weyler was well aware, to match the new prison construction programs being carried out in the other older states in the East. Ours, he wrote, "is one of the few which has held on to its antiquated Penitentiary buildings for generations, merely adding one cell house after another, with the multiplication of prisoners until to-day she has in one pile of bricks, three dormitories patched together in an unsightly heap, one reared against and overlapping the other, and shutting out effectively those elements so essential to health—light and pure air. . . . Further patchwork will only be a waste of money."[24] He urged the immediate construction of a new penitentiary with modern cell houses, to be designed by Baltimore architect Jackson C. Gott.[25]

At its 1890 session the assembly already had appropriated a sum of $250,000 for the enlargement of the penitentiary northward from the upper yard to Eager Street, but the money was to be doled out in installments of only $25,000 per year for ten years.[26] In response to Weyler's urgent appeals, the legislators in 1892 doubled the payments to $50,000 per year, thereby cutting in half the time needed for the building program.[27]

Ground was broken for the new penitentiary buildings in 1894.[28] Two years later the large square administration building, centerpiece of the new complex, was completed, but not its two dormitory wings. Three years later the west (Eager Street) and south (Forrest Street) wings were also in place, though the latter wing stopped at only one-quarter of its planned length to Madison Street, probably because funds ran short. On December 10, 1899, the prisoners moved into their new cell houses. Weyler closely supervised the transferal, which took place without incident. At 10 A.M., 816 prisoners were assembled in the dining room, wearing tags with their new cell numbers and clutching their bundles of

[23]*Board of Directors Report* (1889), pp. 9, 12. Nearly a hundred years later, some of the blocks remain in place after a contractor making renovations lost money trying to remove them. (Interview with Captain William Jednorski, Maryland Penitentiary, November 4, 1987.)

[24]*Board of Directors Report* (1893), pp. 10–11. For a summary of the new prison construction programs in the other eastern states, see McKelvey, *American Prisons,* pp. 176–82.

[25]Jackson C. Gott (1828–1909), F.A.I.A., was a lifelong citizen of Baltimore, who planned both public and private buildings, among them the Johnson Building on North Howard Street and a structure for the Crown Cork and Seal Company at Highlandtown. See Henry F. Withey, *Biographical Dictionary of American Architects (Deceased)* (Los Angeles, Calif.: New Age Publishing Co., 1956), p. 242. Withey strangely omits Gott's most conspicuous achievement, the new Maryland Penitentiary.

[26]*Laws of the State of Maryland* (1890), chaps. 200 and 202, pp. 217, 229.

[27]In the *Board of Directors Report* (1892), Weyler thanked the assembly for speeding up the payment of the appropriated money, as well as for following his recommendations regarding the transfer of insane convicts to asylums in the area and adoption of the (then) new Bertillon system of identifying habitual criminals (p. 14).

[28]*Board of Directors Report* (1899), p. 25.

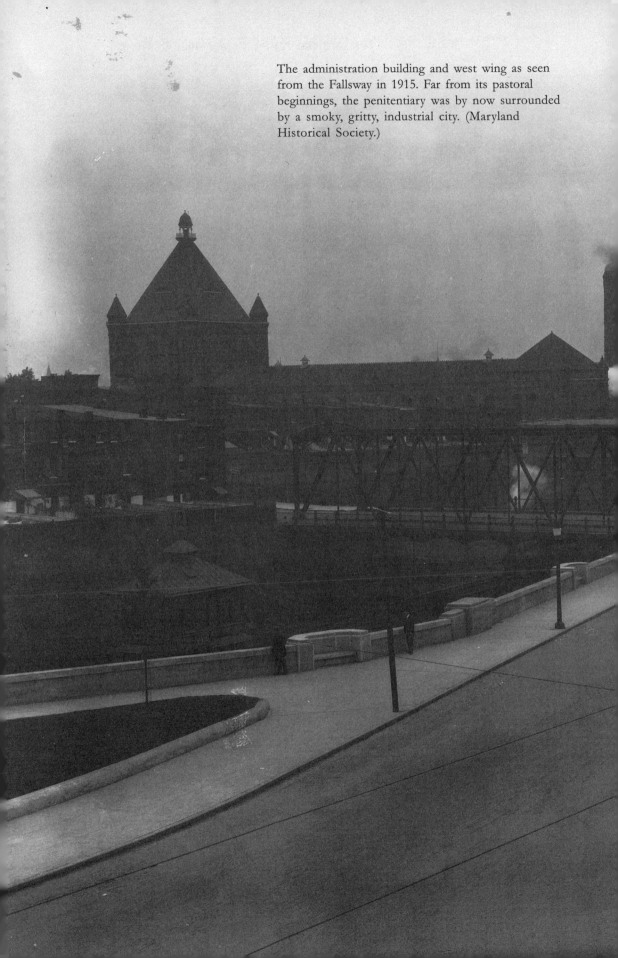

The administration building and west wing as seen from the Fallsway in 1915. Far from its pastoral beginnings, the penitentiary was by now surrounded by a smoky, gritty, industrial city. (Maryland Historical Society.)

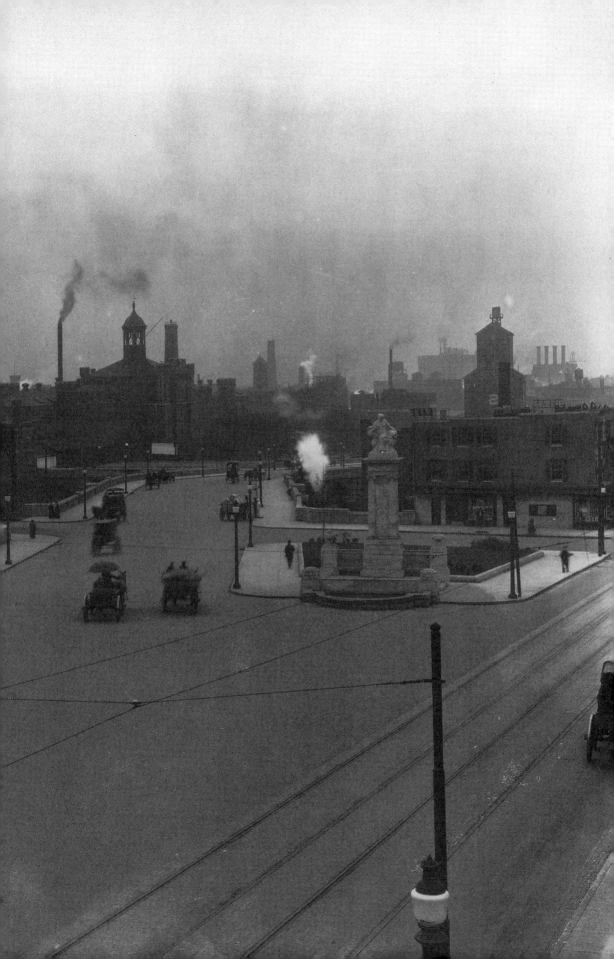

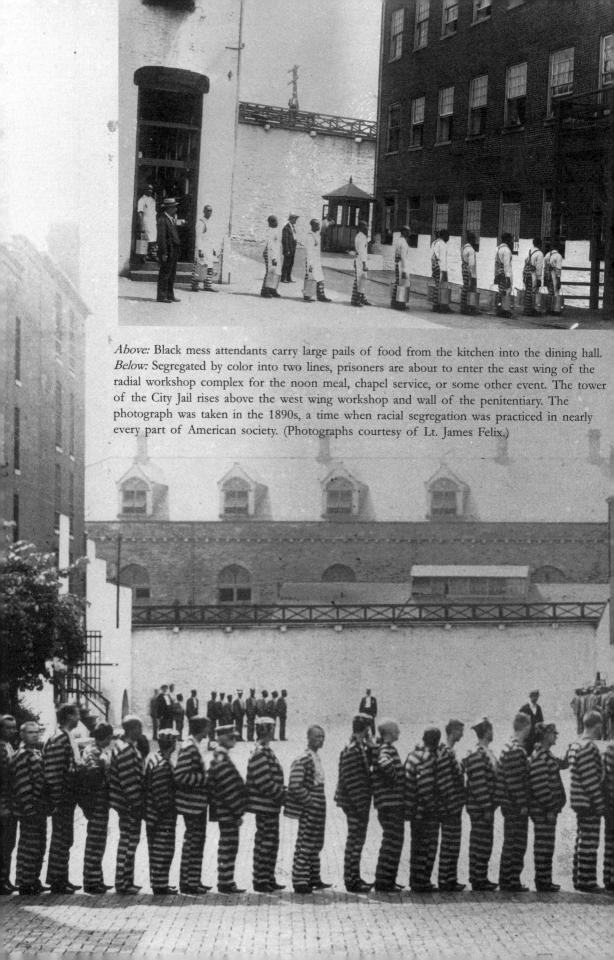

Above: Black mess attendants carry large pails of food from the kitchen into the dining hall. *Below:* Segregated by color into two lines, prisoners are about to enter the east wing of the radial workshop complex for the noon meal, chapel service, or some other event. The tower of the City Jail rises above the west wing workshop and wall of the penitentiary. The photograph was taken in the 1890s, a time when racial segregation was practiced in nearly every part of American society. (Photographs courtesy of Lt. James Felix.)

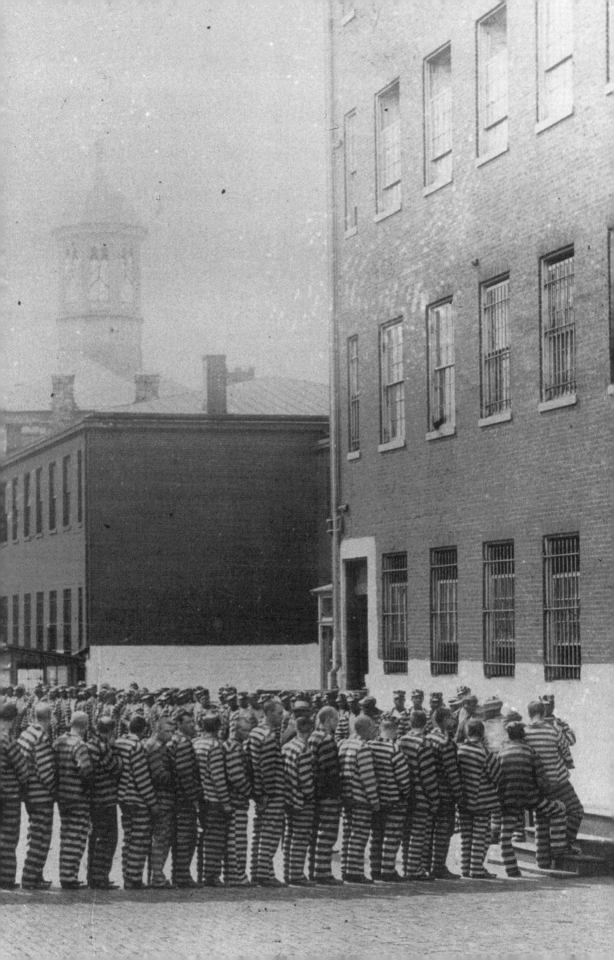

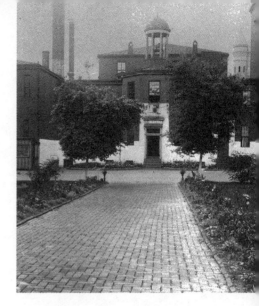

Right: This photograph, taken during the Weyler investigation, shows the octagonal keeper's office with its cupola and dinner bell and the inspection corridors leading into adjoining workshop wings. A tower-like corner of the new administration building rises upper right between the north and east wings of the workshop complex. (Courtesy, Lt. James Felix.)

Below: New dining hall (1899). The men all sat facing one in direction, to discourage conversation. Food consisted of stew, mush, or soup, requiring only spoons, which were picked up at the door and returned on the way out. (Maryland Historical Society.)

Opposite: A page from the penitentiary's prisoner reception book for 1900 shows that techniques for identification have become more complex since the vague "several natural marks on the breast" that identified the first inmate, "Negro Bob" Butler. (Courtesy, Maryland Division of Correction.)

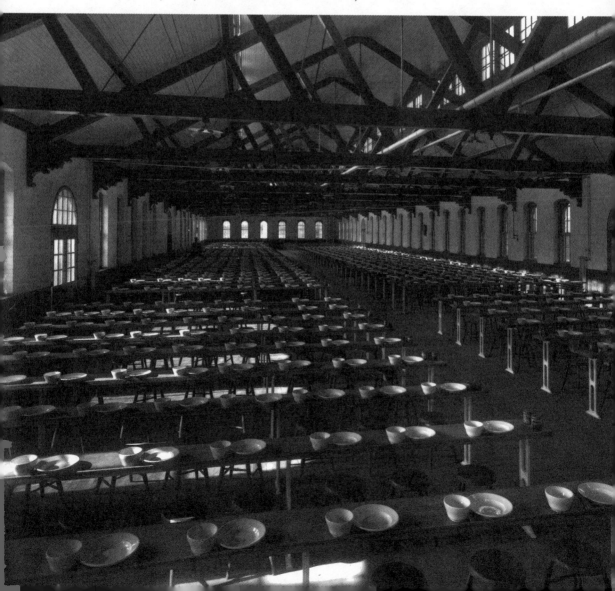

15428

When Received, February 20th 1900
Name, John Washingfield
Where Born, Baltimore Md
Age, 22 Years
Complexion, White
Hair, Light
Eyes, Blue
Stature, 5 foot-8½ inches 168 lbs
Place of Residence, #1211 Plum Alley Balto Md
Occupation, Driver
Marks, Scars top & side of head, Large red mole top of right collar bone, 2 brown moles left side, Brown mole left shoulder back, Large brown mole top of right shoulder, 3 moles abdomen front, Tattooed figures of Buffalo Bill, anchor, Horse head, cannon & flag, Eagle & shield, star & cross, also forming a bracelet across left arm and wrist, Tattooed U & I, Male & Female figures on back of left hand, Tattooed Ivy on left middle finger, Tattooed cross anchor & heart, J.W., Base Ball Player with bat, Pick & letters dig out Gunner, Bird with branch, Female Juggler on right arm, shield & eggs on back of right hand & wrist, star on right wrist, Flags & Shield on abdomen front Sign Board & towels keep off the grass and flying bird below navel, Female leg on left leg, J. H. L & G on right leg lower,

Baltimore City Court—

15429

When Received, February 20th 1900
Name, Randolph Williams
Where Born, Baltimore Md
Age, 24 Years
Complexion, Black
Hair, Wooley
Eyes, Hazel
Stature, 5 foot-7 inches 143 lbs
Place of Residence, #755 George Street-Balto. Md.
Occupation, Waiter
Marks, Scars left side of head, 3 dull scars center of Column back, Birth mark on right collar bone, Tattooed Anchor & heart-right forearm front, Small round head, Short narrow face, Nose long & pointed, Small mouth & lips, chin narrow, Ears Small & set close, Light brown skin, Medium built—

Baltimore City Court—

15430

When Received, February 23rd 1900
Name, Ernest Lehman
Where Born, Baltimore City
Age, 42 Years
Complexion, White
Hair, Black
Eyes, Gray
Stature, 5 foot-8½ inches 148 lbs
Place of Residence, #633 West Lee Street-Balto Md
Occupation, Painter
Marks, Scar under left side of chin, Adams apple prominent mole on chest front, Mole back of neck, Hairy mole base of Column right side Narrow face, long nose, Short chin, Ears large prominent & prolonged, Sallow Complexion, Slender built—

Baltimore City Court—

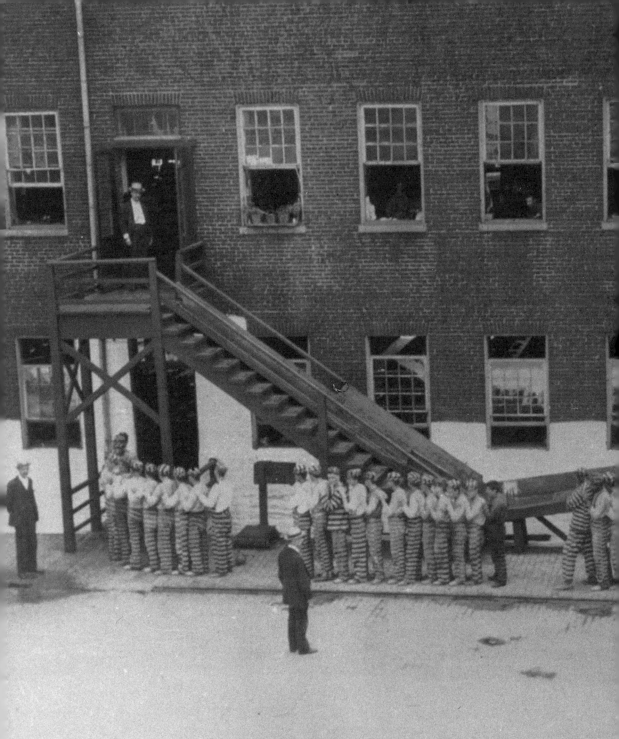

The noon "feed-up" ca. 1895. Here prisoners are formed up in segregated groups of manageable size, ready to move inside the east wing of the radial workshop complex under the watchful eyes of straw-hatted guards. Inmates wore the coarse woolen striped clothing winter and summer. Note that the guards did not wear uniforms. (Courtesy, Lt. James Felix.)

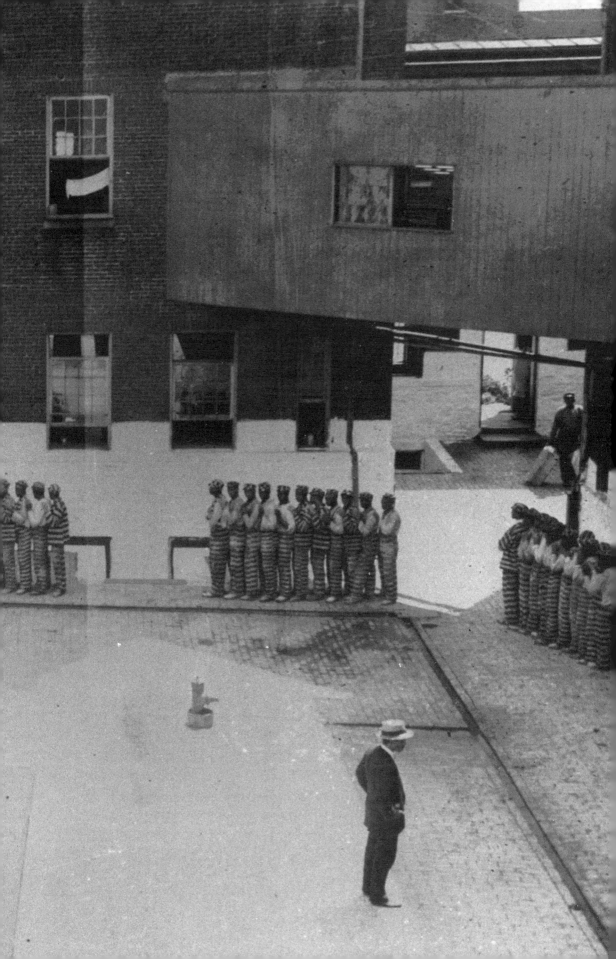

possessions. On command they marched silently across the yard in lockstep, left hands on the shoulders of the men in front, looking in their striped suits "like a waving mass of black and white bars." Little more than an hour later they were locked in their new cells, "delighted with the conveniences."[29]

Today a person looking at the grim castle-like structure, dark with the ingrained soot and dirt of nearly a century, might not believe it was once the subject of civic pride and grandiose language. Costing slightly more than a million dollars, the new penitentiary was hailed as a "massive and handsome structure" that would stand for all time as an "imperishable monument to the humanitarianism of the State." Its main features included the imposing central administration building, constructed in Romanesque style of Port Deposit granite, rising four stories, with a three-story warden's residence on the Eager Street side. Blocks of cells—540 in the Eager Street wing and 280 cells in the Forrest Street wing—were constructed as interior steel cages unattached to the exterior walls ("a prison within a prison, . . . [which] makes escapes practically impossible") with enclosed balconies ("to prevent insane or dangerous prisoners from jumping over or throwing the turnkey from the upper stories"). Sliding cell doors replaced the old-style hinged doors, and the cells were lighted, well ventilated, and larger (nine feet long by five and a half feet wide by eight feet high), each furnished with a large folding bunk and—for the first time in any penitentiary—a combination enameled lavatory and flush toilet ("without crevice or crack to harbor germs") to replace the old "filth" bucket.[30] The new penitentiary's steel and granite construction supposedly ensured against fire, vermin, and escapes. A new two-story power house, built of granite in the same architectural style as the other new buildings, provided steam heat and electric power for the entire institution. A large one-story dining hall, built of brick, seated 1,050.[31]

The year 1899 proved to be Weyler's banner year, for besides the opening of this modern penitentiary, the *Annual Report* declared the largest surplus ever paid into the state treasury ($35,185.34) and the largest amount ($24,884.54) convicts ever earned for themselves through contract "overwork." The prison

---

[29]*Baltimore Sun,* December 11, 1899.

[30]McKelvey, *American Prisons,* p. 181. While an undoubted improvement over the old "filth" buckets, these flush toilets would prove a source of future trouble. Rebellious prisoners could stop up the toilets and flood their cells and adjoining walkways on each tier. Over the years, the steel framing of the walkways in the south wing (used for segregation of unruly inmates) became badly rusted and no longer able to support the heavy slate slabs of the walkways. In the fall of 1988, three slabs on a third tier walkway broke through their rusted steel framing and fell to the tier below, a structural failure brought on by inmates purposely "jumping up and down in cadence, creating additional stress" (*Baltimore Sun,* November 3, 1988).

[31]*Board of Directors Report* (1899), pp. 20–38, 40–41, 43.

board of directors credited his "untiring efforts" toward completion of the new penitentiary and wrote that his "splendid executive work entitles him to the praise of the people of our State."[32]

As large annual surpluses continued to roll in, the directors became increasingly effusive in their praise. "The reputation of the institution, both at home and abroad, speaks volumes for his management, which it is our pleasure to endorse," they declared in 1901.[33] Five years later, they paid tribute to Weyler's "exceptional skill, ability, and fidelity" and reported that despite his strict discipline and rigid economy, he "enjoys not only the respect and affection of his entire official family but the genuine love of the prisoners themselves." As evidence of the convicts' affection, the directors reprinted a description of the transfer of seven federal prisoners from Baltimore to Atlanta. They had bade goodbye to Weyler "with tears streaming down their cheeks," the newspaper observed. "Nor was the usually stern Warden unaffected." After a brief farewell speech, Weyler extended his hand to each of the seven men then "turned away and, shoving his hands into his trousers pockets, walked to the window. Evidently he had a bad cold, for his eyes filled and he was obliged to use his handkerchief; and the cold must have affected his voice, for it was husky when he said another goodbye in reply to the broken goodbyes of the two colored and four white prisoners."[34]

A crescendo of praise came in 1911, which marked both the centennial of the penitentiary and Weyler's last full year as warden. Paying tribute to Weyler's twenty-four-year reign, the directors happily noted the near equality of the total surplus paid to the state ($547,918.70) and the total sum earned by the prisoners for themselves ($547,503.75) and credited the warden with "the almost scientific adjustment of the rights of both master and servant." Calling his administration "phenomenally successful" and citing his international reputation and "the indisputable fact that he has converted the Maryland Penitentiary into a model reformatory rather than a penal institution," the board recommended a special legislative enactment to retain Weyler after his impending retirement with the title of warden emeritus and a yearly salary of $3,000.[35]

The story of Weyler's retirement—really semi-retirement—clearly showed the extent of his power. He had handpicked the new warden, his assistant John F. Leonard. All other promotions or re-appointments of officers and employees followed the recommendations of the warden emeritus. In addition to the honorific

---

[32]Ibid., pp. 12, 6–7

[33]*Board of Directors Report* (1901), p. 5.

[34]*Board of Directors Report* (1906), pp. 6–8.

[35]*Board of Directors Report* (1911), pp. 6–7.

title he would hold the key position of purchasing agent with an annual salary of $3,000—$1,000 higher than that of the new warden.[36] At a testimonial ceremony he received a silver punch bowl inscribed with the name of every employee "as a token of affection." During his acceptance speech, his voice "was husky with emotion" and "his eyes were moist."[37]

Only a day before this sentimental scene, a newly hired guard quit at the end of his first day because he could not bear the outcries of three black prisoners being "cuffed up," a punishment in which the prisoner's wrists were handcuffed together and then hauled up by rope until the tips of his shoes just cleared the floor. His story did not surface in the newspapers for nearly a month,[38] at which time an "amused" Weyler read his complaint and called the guard "a coward" for quitting his post.[39] But in the "muckraking" era, the story could not be dismissed so easily. Weyler became sufficiently concerned about aroused public opinion to write a special report (undated, but written sometime in June) to the prison board defending his disciplinary methods and revealing racial attitudes widespread at the time. "Two-thirds of the inmates here are negroes, and many of these of the so-called Border-State type, confessedly the most difficult to handle and keep in subjection when confined," he claimed. "It is seldom that a plain talk with a white prisoner is ineffectual, but there are colored men—the class that generally comes here—who cannot be made to understand anything unless it is beaten into them." Soon afterwards, in July, Governor Phillips Lee Goldsborough appointed a three-man commission to investigate "the methods of punishment and employment of convicts and the general administration of the Penitentiary."[40]

In charge of the inquiry was Eugene O'Dunne, a young lawyer filled with the reforming zeal of the Progressive Era.[41] Born on June 22, 1875, O'Dunne

---

[36]To Weyler's credit, as his own retirement approached, he carefully groomed Leonard for the job over a two-year period, thus ensuring a smooth change of command (*Baltimore Sun*, May 2, 1912). He had known Leonard at least from the time of their service together on the city council (*Officers of the Corporation*, 1888, p. 6).

[37]*Baltimore Sun*, May 1, 1912.

[38]The ex-guard, Harley Warfield, age forty, had gone back to oystering on the Eastern Shore. He was finally tracked down by a cub reporter from the *Baltimore News*, which then used his story "to start a crusade for a political housecleaning and correction of the prison's methods of punishment and of handling prison labor." See William Engle, "Torture in the Big House," *Baltimore American*, March 14, 1948, vertical file, Maryland Room, Enoch Pratt Free Library, Baltimore. The editorial policy of the newspaper had been established by former owner Charles H. Grasty, one of Baltimore's leading Progressives. See Crooks, *Politics & Progress*, p. 227.

[39]*Baltimore Sun*, May 26, 1912.

[40]*Penal Commission Report*, p. 3, and Appendix C, pp. 328–29.

[41]O'Dunne's opposition to political machines and bossism is everywhere apparent in his scrapbook and in his unpublished autobiography, "Mr. Jurisprudence" (1938), both owned by his son David O'Dunne of Blue Ridge Summit, Pennsylvania. The first newspaper clipping (*Baltimore Sun*, April 19, 1911) in his scrapbook contained Grasty's remarks on "The Modern Newspaper." Grasty expounded at length on the duty of a newspaper to remain independent of politics and not help the "spoils-hunting and corruption" of "un-

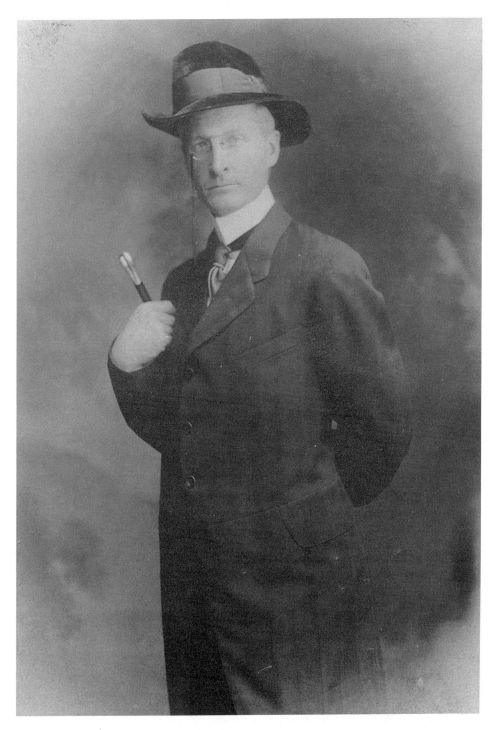

Eugene O'Dunne, a young, reform-minded lawyer, spearheaded the investigation into the penitentiary. H. L. Mencken described him as having "an Irish frenzy to break heads—a kind of boyish delight in alarming sinners and stripping the falsefaces off the virtuous." He is shown here circa 1911. (Courtesy David O'Dunne.)

graduated from the University of Maryland Law School in 1900 and soon after entered public life. Beginning in 1903, he became assistant and then deputy state's attorney, during which time he organized the Young Men's Democratic League and initiated a number of administrative, legal, and judicial reforms. Thereafter, he ran for state's attorney three times unsuccessfully against candidates chosen by the powerful Democratic machine—in 1911, 1915, and 1919. Later, as a judge on the Baltimore City Supreme Bench for nearly twenty years, O'Dunne's caustic wit and colorful antics made frequent headlines. H. L. Mencken described him as seeming to have had "only an Irish frenzy to break heads—a kind of boyish delight in alarming sinners and stripping the falsefaces off the virtuous." But this was only on the surface, he added. "Deep down was a profoundly serious and earnest man—a diligent lawyer, a judge with a tremendous respect for common sense and equal justice." Throughout his long career, the reform-minded O'Dunne fought courageously against vice and corruption and political bossism.[42] Though only half Weyler's age at the time of the investigation, O'Dunne would prove a formidable adversary.

The commission[43] performed its task with thoroughness and dispatch. Along with examining every building and department of the penitentiary, it took nearly fifteen hundred typewritten pages of testimony from prison officials, guards, employees, and contractors. Its members collected more than eight hundred sealed letters from the inmates regarding their treatment, allowing them to voice complaints without fear of reprisal. In addition, the commission sought the opinion of many wardens in the United States and Canada, visited eight other penal institutions, and consulted various leading authorities on prison management.[44] Its report, which appeared only six months after the investigation began, had the usual minor faults of a work produced in haste. Still, it was a

---

clean and dishonorable" party machines and bosses. In his autobiography, O'Dunne told reporters after his first defeat by the Democratic machine candidate in 1911, "What we need in public life today is not so much a new party, as intellectual honesty and intellectual independence" (p. 39). Elsewhere he characterized himself as a "reform judge" (p. 2) and as a person who "did not mix well with the chemistry of organization politics" (p. 73).

[42]See H. H. Walker Lewis, "Baltimore's Judicial Bombshell — Eugene O'Dunne," *American Bar Association Journal,* 56 (1970): 650–55, and O'Dunne's obituary (*Baltimore Evening Sun,* October 30, 1959).

[43]The other two members were Redmond C. Stewart and George L. Jones, described by O'Dunne in his autobiography only as "both citizens of good standing, one a lawyer, the other a social worker" (p. 121). Stewart (1873–1936) received his law degree from the University of Maryland in 1894 and practiced law in the local firm of Stewart & Pearre. See Matthew Page Andrews, *Tercentenary History of Maryland,* 4 vols. (Baltimore: S. J. Clarke Publishing Co., 1925), 2:43–44.

[44]These authorities included Dr. Orlando F. Lewis, General Secretary of the New York Prison Association and the future author of the pioneering historical study *The Development of American Prisons and Prison Customs, 1776–1845* (Prison Association of New York, 1922; repr. Montclair, N.J.: Patterson Smith, 1967).

remarkable document, full of vivid and often unpleasant details, and clearly intended to correct the publicized view of the penitentiary and its management.

At the very outset the penal commission gave credit to Weyler for the erection of the new cellblocks and administration building. But it drew attention to the six "dark" punishment cells in the female department, measuring only four feet wide by eight feet long and eight feet high, without light or ventilation, completely bare except for washbowl and toilet, and closed by a solid steel door with a six-inch by ten-inch opening for food and drink. Moreover, it noted that one hundred male prisoners were still being housed in the dungeon-like cells in the upper four tiers of the old G dormitory, and that the use of the sixty dark punishment cells on the ground tier had been discontinued only shortly after the commission had begun its investigation.

As the commission moved on to criticize the penitentiary's management, its tone sharpened. Contrary to Weyler's statement in his last annual report ("the physical and sanitary condition of the entire Institution is almost perfect in every particular"), the commission found the cells throughout the penitentiary to be generally filthy and infested with bedbugs everywhere, including the male and female hospital wards. "On some of the mattresses of the cells . . . hardly a square foot of ticking presented a surface free from the stains of blood from bedbugs." Sanitary conditions in the ancient G dormitory were "almost past belief"; the men undergoing punishment in the ground tier dark cells slept only on boards infested with bedbugs and covered underneath with cobwebs and white rows of bedbug eggs. And the man in charge, Officer Buckley, admitted, "There are rats all through the place." The sealed letters handed in by the prisoners abounded with angry complaints about the food, from which the commission later offered excerpts. One letter writer called the prison fare "vile and utterly unfit for human consumption." Another wrote, "The meat at most times had a bad smell so as to turn any man's stomach." Still another said, "This morning, Aug. 31, 1912, the breakfast was so bad that the men could not eat it, and the Warden [Leonard] came around [to] the shops distributing bread and molasses." One convict wrote, "I have found bugs [in the soup], but not being a naturalist, I cannot describe them with their college titles. I know one for a roach, but . . . [the rest] were just a bug and maggot menagerie in the soup and hash to me." Another letter writer noted some improvement in convict fare since the commission began its investigation and then asked, "Will we have to return to the old bill of fare, after you have finished your investigation?"[45]

On inspecting the kitchen, the commission found live cockroaches in the steam

---

[45] *Penal Commission Report*, pp. 117, 21, 118, 120, 108.

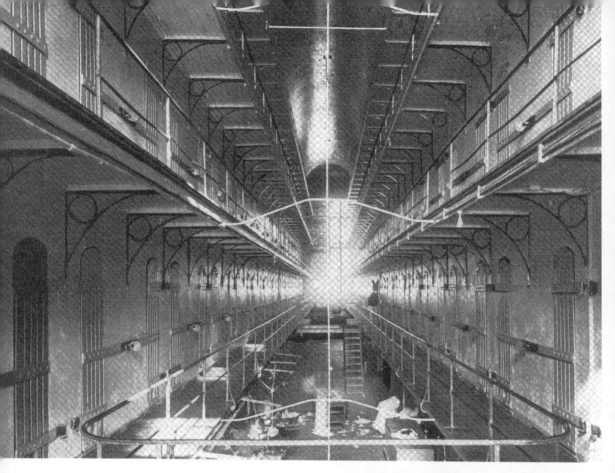

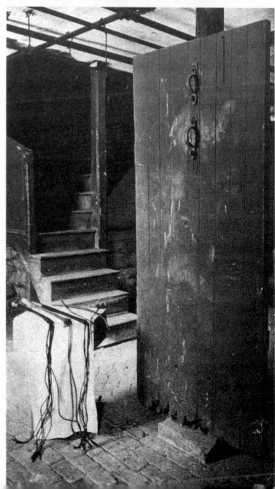

Above: The arcade interior of East Dormitory Wing, designed by Reverend Louis Dwight, president of the Boston Prison Discipline Society, substituted galleries for floors on the upper stories, permitting a single guard to observe every cell, or a preacher to deliver his sermon to all prisoners at once. Though built in 1829, it was still in use in the twentieth century. (From *Maryland Penitentiary Penal Commission Report,* 1913.)

Right: Whipping Board and "Cats." Warden Weyler substituted "cuffing-up" for whipping on the grounds that the latter was unsanitary and contributed to the spread of disease. (From *Maryland Penitentiary Penal Commission Report,* 1913.)

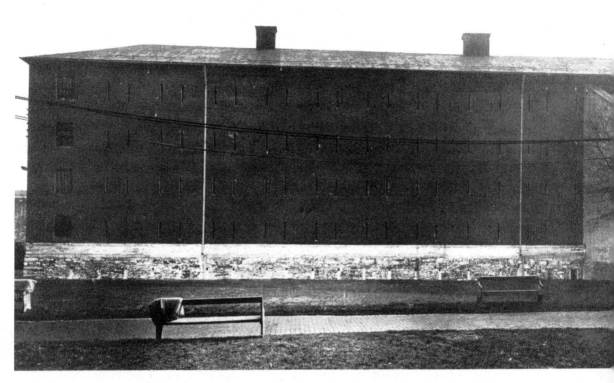

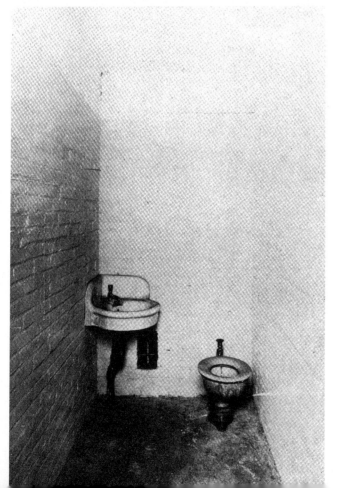

Above: The exterior of old "G" dormitory, showing the six-inch slits for light and ventilation. (From *Maryland Penitentiary Penal Commission Report,* 1913.)

Left: Female punishment cell. Along with other prisons in the nineteenth century, the penitentiary segregated unruly inmates of both sexes in "dark cells," stripped of any furniture. The prisoners were also generally given a reduced diet of bread and water. (From *Maryland Penitentiary Penal Commission Report,* 1913.)

cauldrons, swarms of flies hovering about the uncovered garbage barrels, and no refrigeration for the meat, which soon turned rancid. Asked to identify the beef parts furnished the prisoners, the chief steward, Officer Wollering, admitted he could not distinguish a front leg from a hind leg: "I would have to see it on the cow first."

Censuring the inadequacy of medical care at the penitentiary, the commission noted, among other things, the following: for an average of one thousand inmates, one visiting physician (four hours a day), who endorsed corporal punishment ("cuffing up" or "the cat") to control the insane or feeble-minded; bug-infested hospital beds, having corn husk mattresses; medicines dispensed to the men by a convict pharmacist contrary to regulations; medicines dispensed to the women by the head matron, so ignorant that "she thought antiseptic tablets were strychnine."

The penal commission's heaviest censure of penitentiary management came in the long section on discipline, heralded by a sardonic[46] marginal gloss: "How Sanitation Softened Discipline." Weyler had discontinued the cat-o'-nine-tails six or seven years previously, not because he thought the punishment inhumane but because he believed its use transmitted disease. When "the cat" was laid on a prisoner's back, Weyler explained to the commission, it "of course became saturated with blood of the man, and as . . . [a majority of offenders] are more or less full of syphilis, I considered that to apply that cat to the next man . . . you would open his skin, and necessarily transmit whatever the first man had to the second." Another reason for discontinuing the use of the lash, he said, was that the man's back remained sore for two or three weeks and aroused "a bad spirit."

Weyler had substituted "cuffing up" for whipping as the official form of severe corporal punishment for male inmates, which the commission described in vivid detail: "Handcuffs are fastened on the wrists of the convict, a rope is attached to the chain of the cuffs, then the rope is run over a pipe close to the ceiling, and the offender's hands are drawn up taut above his head. Your Commissioners know from personal experience[47] that the pain caused by a very few minutes of this operation is excruciating." Though prison officials stated that the prisoner was never lifted clear of the ground, almost all the offenders complained about a "third pull" being used: "The first pull extends the man's arms straight above his head; the second drags him up upon his toes or upon the balls of his feet, the third pull swings him clear of the ground." To prevent the offender from climbing the rope and relieving the strain on his wrists, the third pull

---

[46]Written by O'Dunne, who edited the material for publication ("Mr. Jurisprudence," p. 136).
[47]Only O'Dunne had himself cuffed up, "to see how it felt." See "Mr. Jurisprudence," p. 130.

Opposite: "The 'Cuffing-Up' process as arranged by Officer Buckley." (From *Maryland Penal Commission Report,* 1913.)

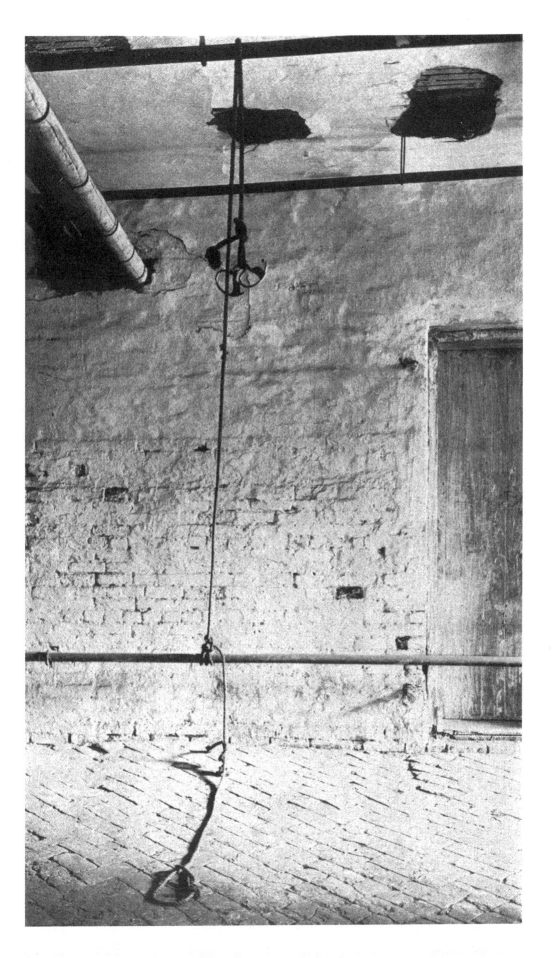

Violation of Rules 1908

Date	Had Up	Task / Cause	Disposition (Total Lost)
Apr. 16	Robt. J. Winston	No Task & Indifference	Cuffed up
" 16	James Glascoe	" " "	" "
" 16	Frank Waters	Breaking pattern	Cautioned
" 17	Wm Bruce	Out of place in line	Cells
17	David Frey	Trading shirt without permission	Lost 60 Days
17	Chas Ward ... Tobe		
18	James Glascoe	Catching iron ahead of bell	Cautioned
20	Wilson Owens	"	Lost 60 Days
20	Wm Satterson	Talking in Dining Room	Cuffed up
20	Oscar Stewart	" "	" "
22	James Robinson ... Shoe	" "	Cells before supper
22	Chas Sanford Shoe	" "	
23	Wm A. Crutchfield	Smuggling meat out of Dining-Room	Cuffed up
24	Richard Brady	Catching iron ahead of bell	Cautioned
24	James Brown #1	"	"
24	James Carroll #1	Talking in Dining Room	"
25	Geo Johnson #1	Talking & not keeping in line	Cells
25	Wilson Owens	Loud talking in shop & Profane Language	"
25	Chas Dennis	Short List & Catching iron ahead of bell	Cuffed up & 60 days
25	James Glascoe	Breaking pattern	Fined $1.50
28	Wm Giles	Catching iron ahead of bell	Lost 60 Days
28	John Hamilton		
29	James Fry	Short List	Cuffed up
30	Allen Manokey	Out of place in line & Impudence	Reprimand
30	Chas. Easton	Catching iron ahead of bell	Cautioned
30	David Burnes	" " " "	"
30	Eugene Roberts	" " "	"
30	Wm Thurman	Fighting in shop	Cells
30	Jos. McClennan Gross	" "	"
May 1	Chas. Dennis	Short List	Cuffed up
" 1	Wm Cornish	"	Cautioned

was most frequently inflicted by tying a rope to the man's ankles and attaching it to a nearby radiator pipe, thus leaving him suspended by his wrists and ankles— for as long as thirty to forty-five minutes, according to an admission by Officer Buckley, the guard in charge of cuffing up.

The system of contract labor at the penitentiary, like that of its discipline, drew heavy censure from the commission. At the outset, it exonerated Weyler of accusations that he suppressed competition in the awarding of contracts and leased out convict labor at less than the going rate. Indeed, it paid tribute to Weyler's efficiency, saying that during his twenty-four years of management, the penitentiary had stopped operating at a loss and had become "a highly organized money-making machine" that returned large annual surpluses to the state. But the state should not allow this to be done, the commission argued, by abandoning its obligation to rehabilitate its convicts: in leasing out their labor to private business firms, the state transfers its control to individuals naturally intent on obtaining cash profit with "no regard for the mental, moral or physical health of the prisoners." The contractor's employees in the penitentiary's shops were "solely interested in driving the convicts to the utmost limit." The prison guards assigned to the shops were their allies, as shown by the contractors' common practice of giving Christmas gifts (usually a $15 gold piece) to each man. Indeed, the commission said, "the brutal and immoderate discipline at the Maryland Penitentiary may be fairly attributed to a desire to drive the convicts to nerve-wracking and excessive labor," as evidenced by the punishment records listing men cuffed up "with almost monotonous regularity" for failing to perform their assigned task.

The commission proceeded to demolish Warden Weyler's defense of the contract system. First it examined his claim that the system yielded to the prisoners themselves an amount equal to the surplus paid to the state. Not only had Weyler "greatly exaggerated" their earnings, it said, but he had also presented "a totally false impression" of their financial benefit to the prisoners. As a case in point, the commission presented the testimony of the foundry's top earner, black convict Sidney Johnson. Under questioning by Chairman O'Dunne, Johnson revealed that he averaged $50 per month, but had to pay out $30 in "expenses"— for foundry helpers, for example, or for chewing tobacco to bribe the kitchen convict to steal extra food so he could get through the heavy work at the foundry. "I have worked out there," Johnson told the commissioners, "until the blood would run out of my hands. You know I was in awful shape when Warden Weyler had to send and get me a pair of gloves to work with. My hands were broken open clean to the bone and blood would come out and sand would get in there . . . and you have no idea how I would suffer with my hands." Weyler had used Johnson, the "star man" in the foundry, as his "chief advertising medium" for

Opposite: A page from the Rules Violation Record of 1908 documents the harsh punishment of "cuffing up." (Photograph by Alan Scherr. Courtesy Maryland Division of Correction.)

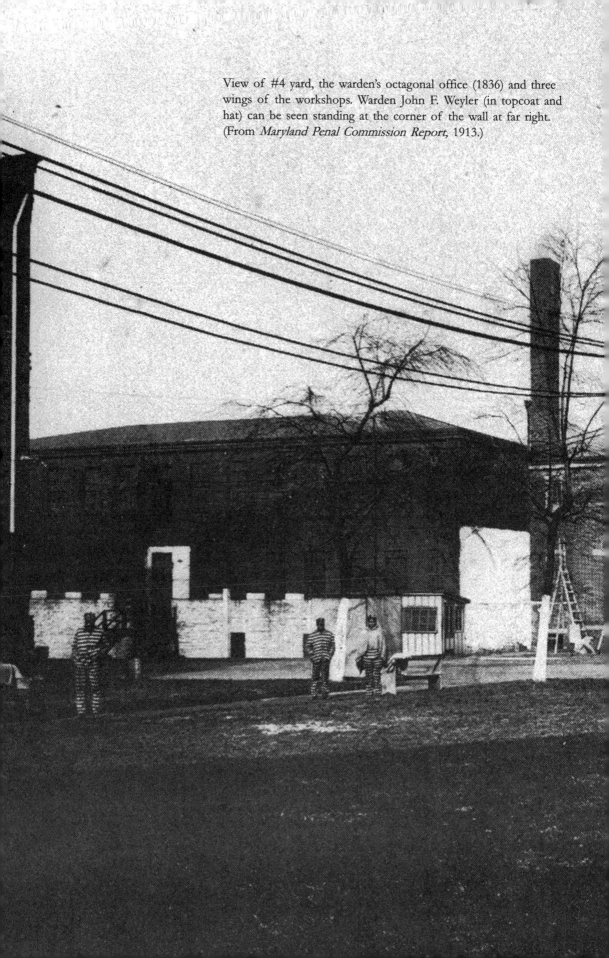

View of #4 yard, the warden's octagonal office (1836) and three wings of the workshops. Warden John F. Weyler (in topcoat and hat) can be seen standing at the corner of the wall at far right. (From *Maryland Penal Commission Report*, 1913.)

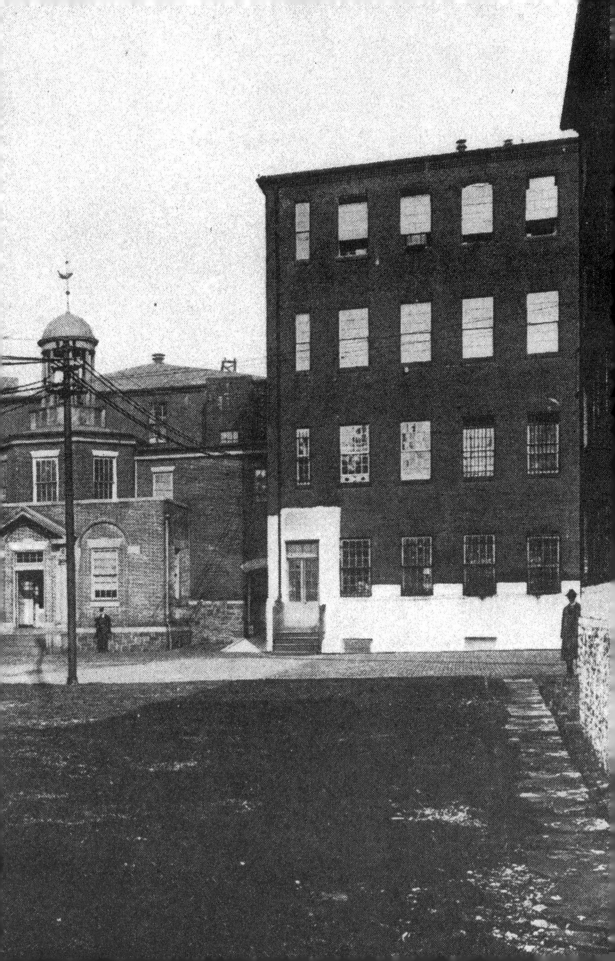

the contract labor system whenever the grand jury visited the penitentiary and had even coached him before he talked to one investigative reporter.

The commission next pointed out the inequities of the contract labor system, when many convicts made little or nothing at all because of the particular kind of work assigned to them. Finally, it examined Weyler's contention that the contract labor system enabled "a very great majority" of discharged convicts to leave the penitentiary with "substantial sums" ($100 or $200) in their pockets that helped them get started in a better life. The commission found instead that of the 431 men discharged in 1911 (the year chosen by Weyler himself), 67 percent had less than $10 to their credit. Weyler had "willfully garbled the records" and was guilty of "deliberate misrepresentation." In conclusion, "The culminating vice of the contract system is that it inevitably induces a money-making spirit on the part of the Warden." And although the commission did not mention Weyler by name, it clearly had the contract system's chief defender and advocate in mind when it spoke of how the prisoners suffered in their bodies and minds when the warden sought "the public applause that comes from turning a money surplus into the Treasury of the State." This same profit motive, the commission implied later, led Weyler to influence his colleagues on a special commission in 1906 to reject the proposed rehabilitative plan of the indeterminate sentence and its concomitant, the parole system, because it would interfere with the steady supply of convict labor in the shops.[48]

Although the penal commission found no evidence to show that Weyler took any money for himself from the contract labor system, it had aired a possible motive for his defense of that system: a thirst for "public applause" or prestige. Another possible motive—the satisfaction in manipulating people and events—emerged in the story of his collusion with the contractors at the penitentiary. Asked by Chairman O'Dunne about his part in helping to defeat anti-contract labor legislation in Congress in 1900, Weyler testified on September 14, 1912, that acting as a member of a prison lobby, he paid $2,500 from their fund to hire the law firm of Dudley & Michener to work against the bill. When the bill passed the House and went to the Senate, he obtained the help of his old political friend, former Senator Gorman, who gave it "wholly as a friendly matter and without one cent of compensation" and the bill was subsequently pigeon-holed. Pressed by O'Dunne for further details, Weyler admitted to having paid $4,000 to an undisclosed party for help in the anti-prison labor fight. With still more prodding, he gave the other attorney's name: Arthur Pue Gorman Jr., son of the former Senator.

---

[48] *Penal Commission Report*, pp. 208, 212, 216.

When the commission arrived at young Gorman's office the next morning, it discovered that Weyler had departed only minutes before. Through personal interviews and correspondence with Gorman, Chairman O'Dunne then tried repeatedly to obtain further information but ran into a stone wall. Gorman claimed he could not remember details about the eleven-year-old transactions and that the records probably had been destroyed in the great Baltimore fire of 1904. He admitted receiving a fee of $4,000 from Weyler but haughtily denied kicking back any of it to him, "as neither myself nor the firm . . . found it necessary to obtain clients in such a manner." He denied that his father had had anything to do with defeating the anti-prison labor bill.

Here the commission paused to characterize Weyler's testimony thus far as "dissembling . . . grossly deceptive . . . misleading . . . artful and elusive," and added yet another illustration: his emphatic denial of any knowledge of Christmas gifts presented by the contractors to the guards assigned to their shops. But according to the shirt contractor, "It was done openly . . . for eleven years," and the shoe contractor testified, "We could not have turned a wheel without him [Weyler] knowing it."

Weyler had feathered his retirement nest at state expense. On August 16, 1909, toward the end of his long tenure at the prison, he had purchased a sixty-seven-acre farm north of Baltimore near the Timonium fairgrounds.[49] From the time of its purchase, a steady stream of building materials, goods, and services flowed from the penitentiary northward to improve what Weyler proudly called Crystal Farm. First came the 2,800 pounds of discarded radiator piping appropriated by the warden for making fence posts two years or so before the investigation began. When the commission questioned Weyler about this matter on September 14, 1912, it was told immediately after by the prison bookkeeper—to its "utter amazement"—that Weyler had paid him for the piping less than an hour before the interrogation. Although later questioned relentlessly by the young chairman about his cover-up, Weyler denied any wrongdoing. The warden also had appropriated the services of the penitentiary's engineer, former convict Frank Hare, who had gone out to the farm on several occasions and worked on both the windmill and the greenhouse. Summoned to testify before the commission at the penitentiary the same day as Weyler, September 14, Hare called in sick. The commission subsequently discovered that the supposedly sick man conferred with the warden at his farm the very next day, at which time he was paid for the work done there in the past.

The warden's alleged appropriation of penitentiary food waste—especially bread

---

[49]Court Record 30,747, deed #410, folio 365, Maryland State Archives.

Top: Cutting room of the penitentiary's contract workshop. The prison sold prisoners' labor to an outside contractor to help pay for their keep. They could earn additional money for themselves by exceeding their daily "task" or set quota. Sewing was done in the east wing of the radial workshop complex, or G building, which still stands. Beginning in 1916, prison officials phased out the contract system of using prison labor in the face of complaints of unfair competition from free workers. Thereafter prison labor was used to manufacture items for state use, such as furniture and license plates, and, during World War II, uniforms and shoes for the federal government.

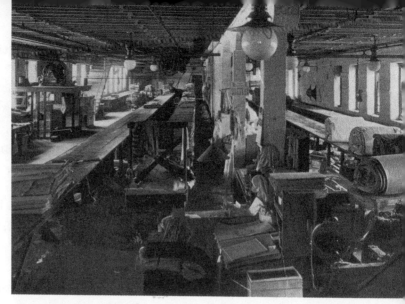

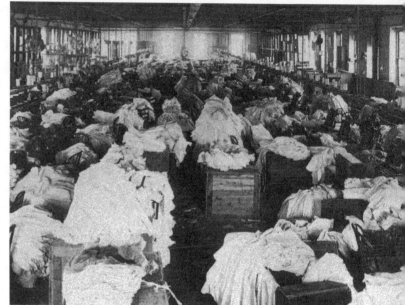

Center: Piles of cloth in cut patterns await sewing into shirts in the workshop's sewing room.

Bottom: The foundry. Note the prisoners' uniforms hanging on the line at right. (From *Maryland Penal Commission Report,* 1913.)

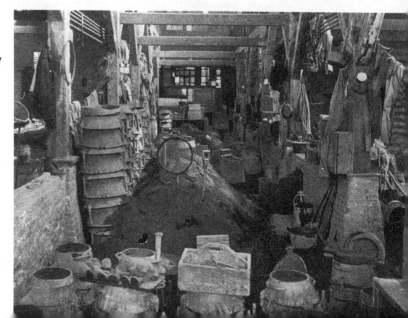

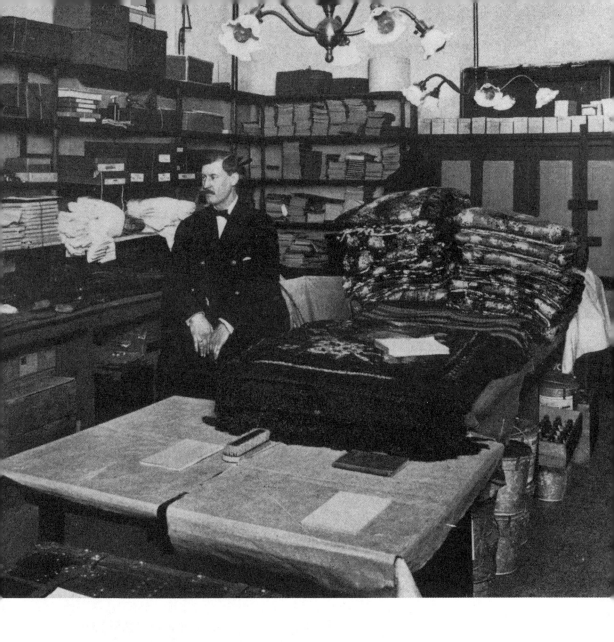

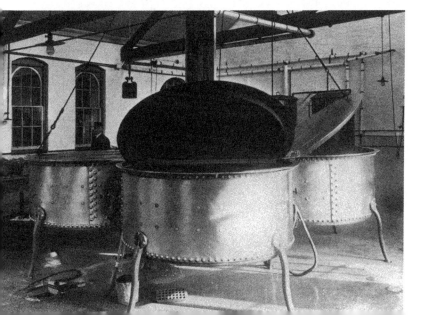

Above: "Mr. Marsh and the Commissary."

Left: Kitchen cauldrons. According to chairman Eugene O'Dunne, "When you put the steam on the roaches run out." (From *Maryland Penal Commission Report*, 1913.)

crumbs for his chickens—proved a large item. Weyler had "habitually" violated sections 556, 596, and 607 of article 27 of the Code of Public General Laws (1904), which prohibited perquisites and required the sale of slop and offal by the institution or their use in raising livestock for the benefit of the prisoners. A meticulously compiled list of railroad waybills showed that from August 12, 1910, to July 26, 1912, he had shipped bags of toasted bread crumbs out to his farm "in quantities ranging from 500 to nearly 3,000 pounds a week," for a total of forty thousand pounds over the two-year period.

Further details of "Weyler's Toasted Bread Industry" came later on September 13, 1912. "The baker puts it in the oven and toasts it. It will mould, you know, if you do not do something to it," the warden's trusty, Charles S. Henry, told the commissioners. "And he browns it up a little. I used to tie the bags up at times. They generally ship on Fridays. At times, there are thirty to fifty bags of bread to go out in one week. . . . This has been going on ever since the damn farm was out there." His testimony made clear that the operation had been halted by Officer Benjamin Kohler, the warden's nephew, shortly after the penal commission began its investigation.

Having risen under Weyler's management to become the penitentiary's "most trusted convict" and its "general handy man," Charles S. Henry knew more than any other inmate about the alleged institutional graft and corruption and proved to be the key witness in the penal commission's investigation. At first he was reluctant to talk, eager to preserve his privileged position and fearful of retribution. "Strange things happen here," he said. But after repeated assurances of protection and immunity by Chairman O'Dunne, Henry at last broke down and told how Weyler had siphoned off manpower and materials from the penitentiary to refurbish his farm.

Working in the penitentiary along with several other convicts, Henry had constructed twenty to twenty-five chicken houses, a duck house, an engine-house, and a greenhouse out of materials appropriated from the stores of contractors and the penitentiary. Engineer Hare was "the main gazook," in charge of the project. Some of the convicts had been "pardoned out" by Weyler to serve as farmhands. According to Henry, engineer Hare would be absent from the penitentiary's powerhouse for days at a time, doing construction work at Weyler's farm. Hare also had a truck built for the farm, the wheels being cast in the foundry and the body made in the yard out of lumber. Henry's recitation of goods and furnishings sent out to the farm lasted until his memory ran dry: chicken crates, kitchen dresser and sinks, radiator piping for the greenhouse, rubber trees, storage boxes, parts for the windmill, tools, wire screens and roofing for the chicken house, leather meat buckets, and a large table made of coffin lumber.

With some further prodding from O'Dunne, the witness agreed to tell the commission the story of graft and corruption inside the penitentiary as well, including his own dealings with its officers. "My God!" he said, "I could write a bookful about it. . . . The whole shooting match is crooked, from beginning to end." At his post in the powerhouse, the trusty took part in Weyler's conspiracy to sabotage the electric plant. "It was a put-up job all the way through to put the Brush Electric Company out of the building and put the Gas Electric Power Company here." Also, as Weyler's "trusty" and therefore able to move freely about the institution, Henry stole shirts, brushes, and other items for the officers and was rewarded with food, daily newspapers, and whiskey. He stole lumber and iron from the foundry for the penitentiary's use while the guards looked on. "The men on the wall . . . saw me coming out of there and they stood there and laughed." From the brush contractor's shop he stole varnish, paint, and turpentine for penitentiary use because his predecessor had "learned" him. "Now Charlie," he said, "if you want to hold this job you go ahead and do as I am doing. Just save all you can for the State and they [the officers] will look out for you." At Christmas time, Henry testified, the inmates were allowed to order groceries, which were delivered a week before distribution and stored in the penitentiary bathroom. "Well, of course those groceries were always short . . . the officers had the key to the bathroom and they would swipe those groceries out of there and then make the grocery man make them good. There was a whole damn wagon load short here once, and the sugar and condensed milk and everything was taken out."

When the penal commission again called Henry to testify four months later, it learned that during the interval he had been deprived of his privileged position as "trusty" and transferred to the shirt shop. "They did not give no excuse," said Henry, and he told the commission how he had been taken out of his comfortably furnished cell, strip-searched, and locked up in the ancient G dormitory. "They said they would get me and they did."

But the commission kept its word and arranged for Henry's pardon, which was delivered January 23, 1913. That same afternoon, Henry, now a free man, repeated for the commission—at chairman O'Dunne's specific request—what assistant engineer Foote (not a convict) had told him upon learning that he (Henry) had testified. "O'Dunne is not nothing. . . . The s— of a b—— ain't no good at all; he could not get elected State's Attorney; he could not get elected for president of a s—house. . . . You will be sorry as soon as you leave because you can not get a job in the City of Baltimore if it is found out that you ever said anything against Weyler."

One last illustration of Weyler's attempts to withhold and suppress evidence

Right: Penitentiaries constantly sought better means of identifying prisoners. These intake records, dating from the Weyler administration, used a combination of photography, the Bertillon measurements, fingerprints, and written physical description. (Courtesy, Maryland Division of Correction.)

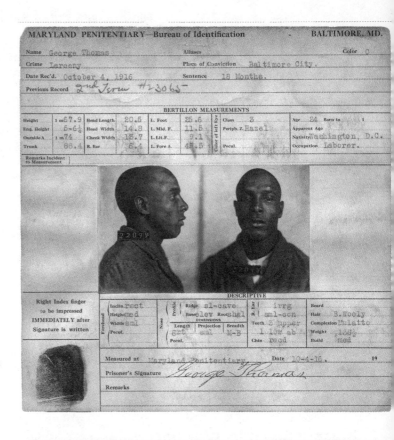

Facing page: The penitentiary's new west wing contained steel cellblocks that were not built into the walls—"a prison within a prison." They also had barred catwalks, so that inmates could not throw themselves, or a turnkey, over the rails. (From *Maryland Penal Commission Report,* 1913.)

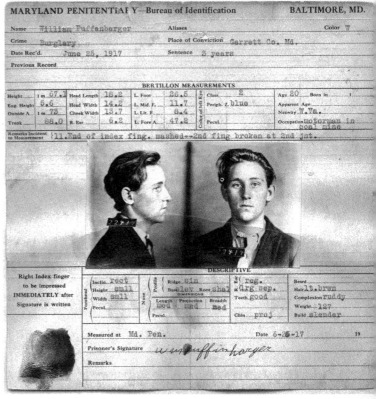

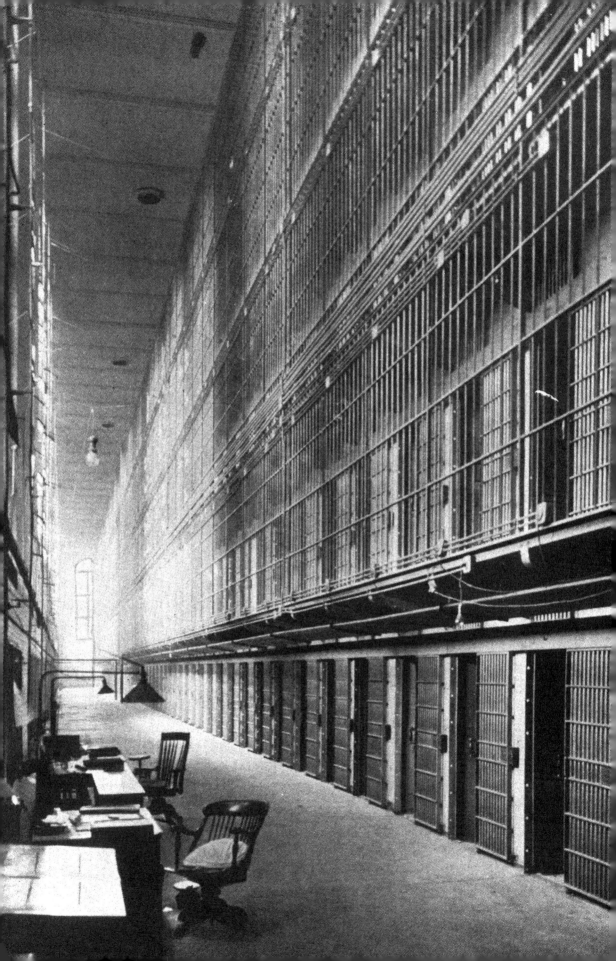

came when Chairman O'Dunne tried unsuccessfully by letter and telephone to obtain an inventory from Weyler of the tools on his farm. Shortly thereafter Weyler's nephew, Officer Benjamin Kohler, admitted reluctantly that, acting at Weyler's request, he had instructed area hardware stores not to furnish the penal commission with copies of the warden's accounts.

The commission delivered a scathing denunciation of the still-powerful warden emeritus, calling him "a man who has not been able to distinguish between property belonging to the State and that belonging to himself, and one on whom truth's virtue rests so lightly." The penitentiary cannot reform its inmates, it said, by setting such a poor example before them. "Owing to his habitual contempt for the provision of statutory law and to the vicious conditions surrounding his administration, the integrity and welfare of the Institution imperatively demand his immediate and final elimination."[50] Weyler's removal proved unnecessary, however. On February 4, 1913, he tendered his resignation to the board of directors, carefully pointing out to them that he had only stayed on until the penal commission had finished examining him, "for any other action I thought might be interpreted as being unmanly, if not cowardly."[51]

Three days later the penal commission filed its completed report with Governor Goldsborough, who immediately released a summary to the press. The story appeared that evening in the *Baltimore Sun* with the sensational headline "PEN PROBERS FLAY WEYLER IN REPORT — Cruelty and Law Violations Are Charged Against Him." While the newspaper account quoted extensively from the report, it omitted the commission's one favorable comment about Weyler's effectiveness in bringing to completion the new penitentiary buildings. The warden's large annual surpluses—his other source of pride—appeared as the product of a man obsessed, achieved at the expense of "the moral, mental, and physical welfare of the convicts." Then came the major reforms recommended by the commission: abolition of the contract labor system, the adoption of the indeterminate sentence and parole for prisoners, and the creation of a central state prison board to oversee all penal institutions, reforms Weyler had opposed but which already had been carried out by the more progressive penal institutions in the nation.[52] The next day was Weyler's sixty-ninth birthday, which "he celebrated . . . by coming to the city . . . and consulting several of his friends in reference to the answer he will make to the commission's report."[53]

---

[50]The *Penal Commission Report* continued for 135 more pages (pp. 206–341): Part VI (pp. 207–24), "The Indeterminate Sentence"; Part VII (pp. 225–30), "General Recommendations"; Part VIII (pp. 231–43), "Summary of Findings and Recommendations"; plus miscellaneous exhibits and appendices.

[51]*Penal Commission Report,* Appendix E, pp. 240–41.

[52]See McKelvey, *American Prisons,* p. 255.

[53]*Baltimore American,* February 9, 1913.

His response, like the penal commission's report, was a remarkable document, but for different reasons. In a thirteen-page statement the former warden presented an artful defense based on the theme of persecution. The report, he said, was aimed at "crushing out the life of an old man who has spent his best years in caring for the unfortunate and in working for the best interests of his native state." The expected "gigantic case of graft" was not found because "John F. Weyler in his conduct of the Maryland Penitentiary for twenty-four years never had his palm tickled by a dishonest dollar." Clearly, Weyler regarded O'Dunne as his personal adversary. He referred to him more than a half-dozen times in the first two pages as "the Chairman" but—as when speaking of the devil—without once mentioning his name. According to Weyler, the chairman had sent private detectives to his farm "to see what loot I had and where I kept it"; had visited the farm himself with a stenographer on a Sunday, while Weyler and his wife were entertaining guests; had sent an agent out to take an inventory of his farm property; had terrorized witnesses with threats of the grand jury; and had granted pardons to witnesses who did testify against him, namely, "Sidney Johnson, colored, a murderer, and Charles S. Henry, white, a horse thief."

After adroitly referring first to his role in the construction of the new penitentiary buildings, to his international reputation as a prison administrator, and to the large annual surpluses turned over by him to the state, he addressed himself to some of the specific charges. The bedbug problem was exaggerated by the report, he said, "though some bedbugs are there and always will be in dormitories of small cells inhabited by 1,000 men, of whom two-thirds are colored persons of the lowest type." Other charges—poor laundry work, rats in G dormitory, lack of proper refrigeration, and bad or inadequate food—he either denied or downplayed. "As to roaches, what hotel kitchen does not have them?"

However, he defended his disciplinary methods at length, claiming that bad conduct "must be nipped in the bud." To illustrate, he cited the case of "a colored convict" whom he ordered lashed (when whipping was still practiced) on two successive days—the first day for misconduct and the second day for coming to his punishment with a concealed knife. From then on, according to Weyler, the offender was a good convict and when discharged "shook my hand and thanked me," saying, "Your treatment has thoroughly reformed me; something that my father tried hard to do and couldn't." The punishment of "cuffing up" was substituted for whipping "for hygienic reasons." Female offenders were punished merely with solitary confinement: "A bad woman, especially a negress, is a worse prisoner than a bad man, because she can maintain her stubborn opposition the longer." No corporal punishment is used on them "because of their sex and the bad ones presume upon it." After dismissing several more

View (ca. 1916) to the southwest from the top of the administration building, showing (lower left) the original, square administration building (1811) now converted to a hospital. The two long buildings to its right are B and C dormitories. Farther to the right is the City Jail. Above its tower, in the background, is the Bromo-Seltzer Tower with bottle, long a Baltimore landmark. (Maryland Historical Society.)

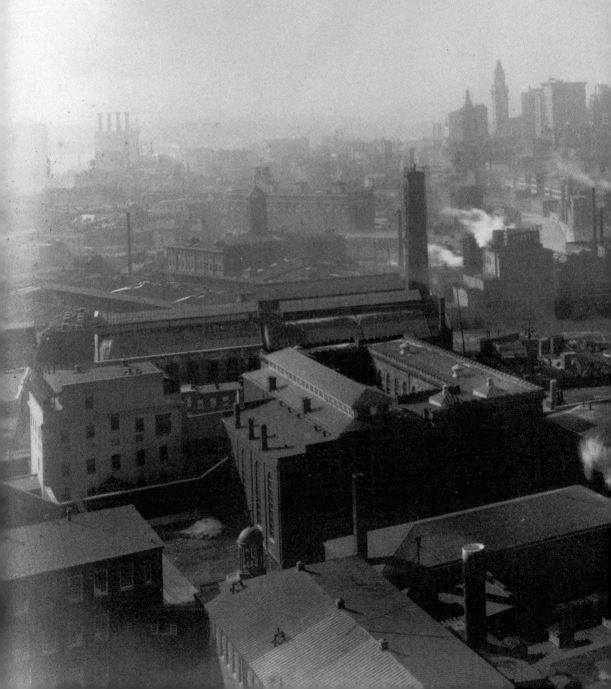

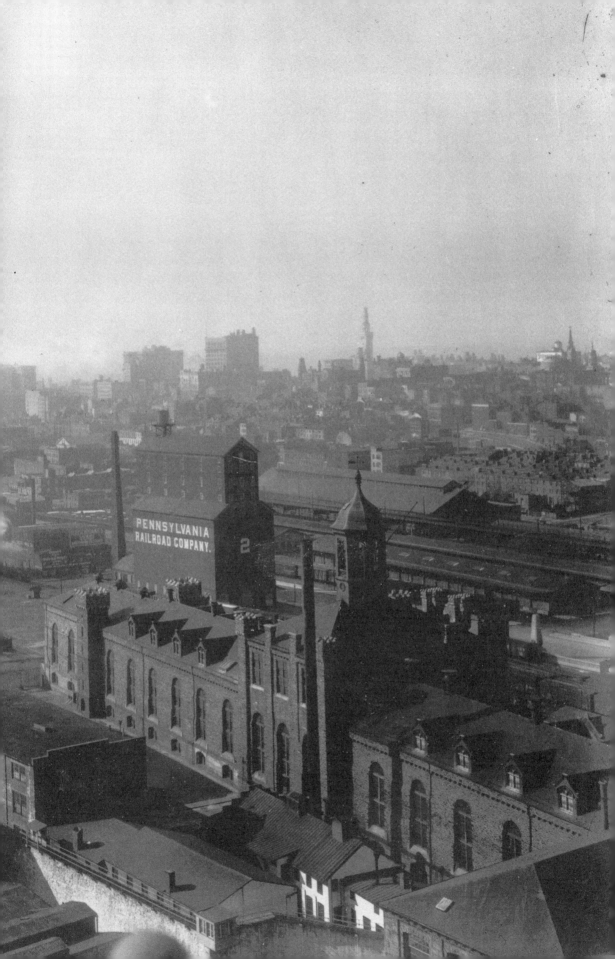

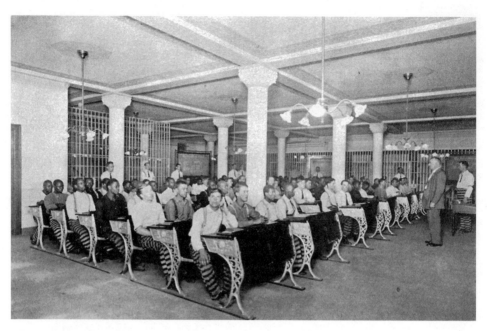

"The School for Male Prisoners." The investigation of 1912 resulted in many reforms. (From *Annual Report,* 1916.)

charges as "utterly groundless," he paused to deliver a rhetorical blast at the penal commission: "How clear it is, then, that they are mistaken in their premises, deluded as to their deductions, warped in their conclusions, utterly unreliable all around and deeply culpable in their pursuit of a man who never tried to do anything but his whole duty." This passage is impressive for its command of language, all the more so considering Weyler's limited formal education. In the final pages, Weyler defended his appropriation of bread crumbs, saying, "I did not believe that it was a crime to save goods of no commercial value. . . . Since the wickedness of it has been made plain to me [by the penal commission], the crumbs go once more into the sewer." His last paragraph returned to the theme of persecution and his (once again) nameless adversary: "One thing is certain. . . . Every act, every query, every inflection of the voice of the chairman of the inquisitors showed to me and others that there was a conviction of me before the trial and that the effort of the inquiry was 'to get Weyler.'"[54]

The penitentiary board of directors, of which Weyler's old friend Frank Furst was president, backed to the hilt Weyler's spirited reply to the charges against him.[55] The board called the O'Dunne report "a sweeping and unqualified arraignment of

[54] *Statements of the Board of Directors of the Maryland Penitentiary and John F. Weyler, Warden Emeritus, In Reply to the Report of Maryland Penitentiary Penal Commission to Hon. Phillips Lee Goldsborough, Governor of Maryland* (Baltimore, 1913), pp. 20–32.

[55] Weyler's letter and the board's statement were published together; see note 54.

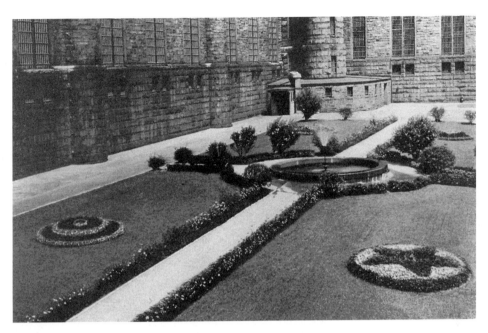

"A Beauty Spot Inside the Walls." The new warden tried to change the image of the penitentiary. (From *Annual Report,* 1916.)

John F. Weyler," based "almost exclusively" on charges made by convicts, thereby depriving Weyler of "a square deal." Members of the penal commission, according to the board, undertook their investigation "with their minds already inflamed, their judgement already warped and with the purpose to apply to their work certain standards and measurements, based upon purely theoretical and sentimental premises." The board then turned to some of the specific charges. "The entire sum of the so-called grafting of Mr. Weyler is trivial," it said, compared to the riches he could have gained by accepting kickbacks from the contractors who employed the convicts. No real graft was found, argued the board. A man with Weyler's opportunities "does not content himself with the petty pilfering of garbage and useless junk"—his use of breadcrumbs and discarded piping and his acceptance of the services of employees and of convicts were "merely improprieties." The board criticized the commission's handling of its convict witnesses, all but accusing its members, and Chairman O'Dunne, in particular, of "the kind of coaching . . . of lawyers who suborn witnesses to commit perjury." Then, like Weyler, the board downplayed the charge of unsanitary conditions at the penitentiary and defended the painful punishment of "cuffing up" as necessary in dealing with the convicts, "many of them . . . desperate characters." In fact, said the board, discipline at the penitentiary was so undermined by the commission's ongoing investigation "that the use of the cat-o'-nine-tails had to be resumed as the only adequate punishment for offenses such as murderous assaults by convicts upon

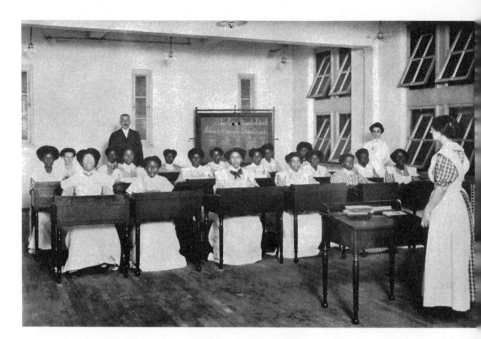

Women's classroom (right) and infirmary (below). (From *Annual Report,* 1916.)

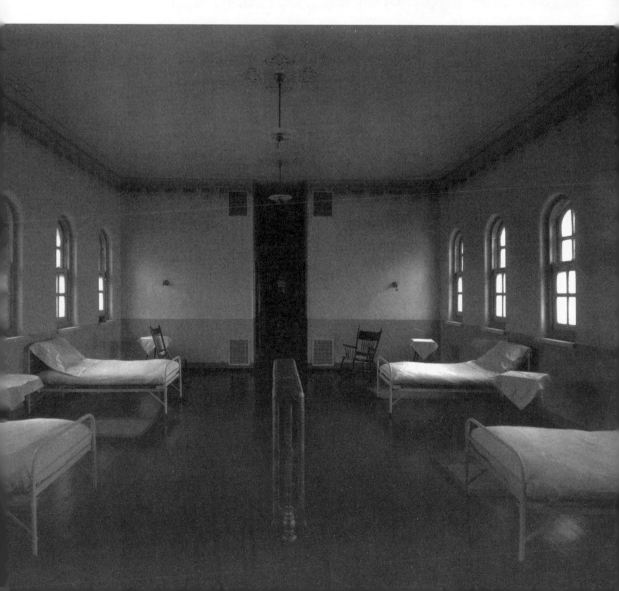

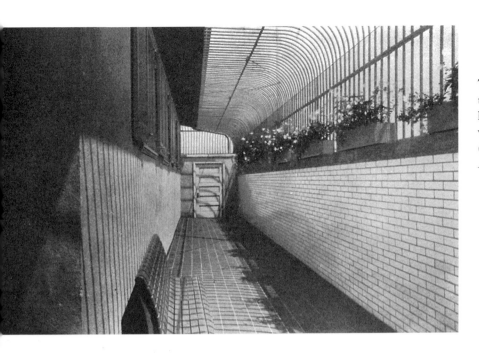

Tubercular ward on the roof of the hospital (left) and women's chapel (below). (From *Annual Report*, 1916.)

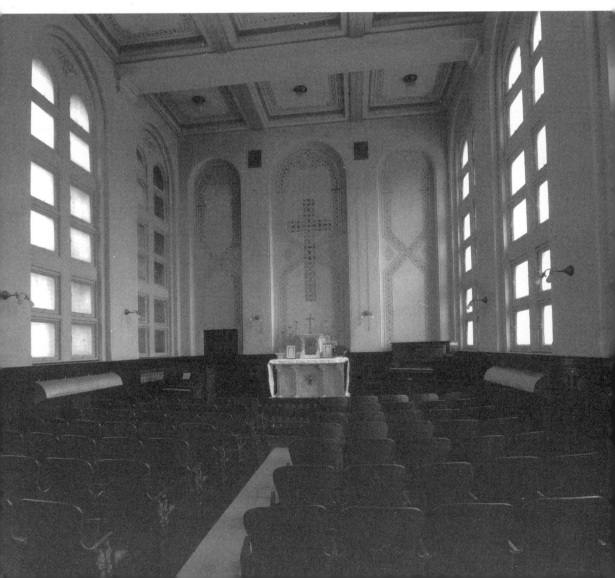

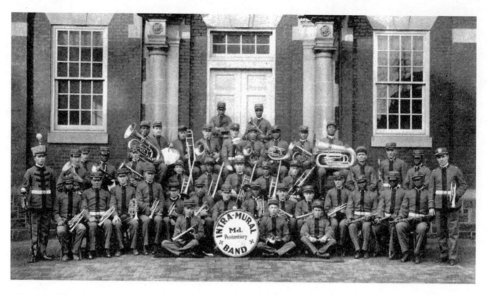

The Maryland Penitentiary band. (From *Annual Report,* 1916.)

guards and fellow convicts."[56] Other charges the board either denied or called matters of opinion. In its concluding statement, the board blamed the penal commission for "setting in the public pillory, labeled with charges of falsehood, graft, and cruelty a faithful public official, who was for more than a score of years at the head of the Maryland Penitentiary."

The local press headlined both the statements of Weyler and of the penitentiary board in a way that surely must have been heartening to the embattled former warden: "PENAL REPORT FLAYED," read one, while another declared somewhat misleadingly, "MR. WEYLER EXONERATED."[57] Only the penitentiary board, of course, had exonerated Weyler. It was the best he could expect, short of an acquittal in a court of law. In fact, Weyler by now had little reason to fear that he would be prosecuted. His departure had already satisfied the commission, and the state's attorney had no evidence that would justify action.[58]

Nevertheless the man once hailed as the penitentiary's "model warden" suffered severely from the O'Dunne commission's charges of mismanagement and cruelty. He lost no time in putting Crystal Farm up for sale, disposing of it in April 1913.[59] Ultimately, he seems to have left Maryland for parts unknown.[60]

---

[56]Although discontinued at the penitentiary later that same year, whipping was still used at the City Jail for wife beaters, in accordance with a law that dated from colonial times and remained in force until April 1953. The last whipping in Maryland took place in Anne Arundel County in 1948. See Harry E. Barnes and Negley K. Teeters, *New Horizons in Criminology* (3rd ed.; Englewood Cliffs, N.J.: Prentice-Hall, 1959), p. 290.

[57]*Baltimore Sun,* March 6, 1913, and *Baltimore American,* March 6, 1913.

[58]*Baltimore American,* February 9, 1913.

[59]Court Records 30,747, deed #410, folio 365, Maryland State Archives.

[60]The Baltimore City Directory for 1914 listed Weyler as living at Walnut and Second Avenues, Rognel Heights (just north of the present-day Edmondson Village Shopping Center). Thereafter he is not to be

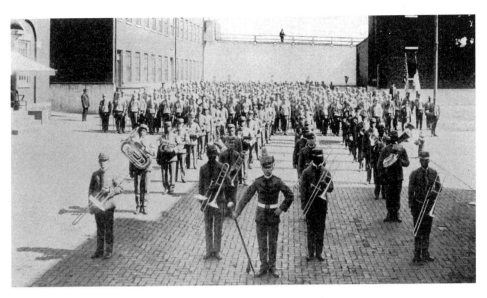

Prisoner musicians taking pride in public drill. (From *Annual Report,* 1916.)

Weyler's career is reminiscent of tragedy and invites a search for a tragic flaw, a somewhat difficult undertaking because of the seventy-five-year interval and because he left behind no personal papers that might reveal his innermost thoughts. Basically, Weyler's flaw seems to have been a craving for power and prestige, which paradoxically was served by an undeniable talent—his administrative skill. He had found the penitentiary in 1888 ailing financially and its buildings in poor condition. Within a few years he had it turning out ever-increasing surpluses and had implemented a building program that resulted in the magnificent granite pile at the corner of Eager and Forrest streets. His success had earned him not only "public applause" but apparently allowed him to dominate the board of directors and become a "king" within the walls of the penitentiary.

His single-minded pursuit of this success, however, apparently led him to resist major prison reforms taking place across the nation.[61] He had not only lobbied against anti-contract labor laws in 1900, but he had fought the rehabilitative plan of the indeterminate sentence and parole system proposed for the penitentiary in 1906 because he believed it would interfere with the steady supply of convict labor in the workshops. Even his alleged cruelty seems to have arisen out of his over-zealous management of the contract labor system at the penitentiary. O'Dunne had paid tribute to Weyler's productivity, but the warden had achieved it through

found in any of the city directories. A search at the Maryland State Archives has turned up no record of his will ever having been probated.

[61]During this period, the movement for the indeterminate sentence and parole for convicts was spreading throughout the country, and by 1915 these reforms had become established in all state prisons except a few in the South. See McKelvey, *American Prisons,* pp. 159, 241, 245–47.

"brutal and immoderate discipline," primarily by "cuffing up" those inmates who failed to perform their assigned daily task, as extensively documented in the prison's punishment records.[62] Weyler, then, appears to have regarded the inmates merely as objects to be manipulated, as cogs in his penitentiary machine. Here it is important to remember that he had substituted the punishment of "cuffing up" for whipping not for humane but for practical reasons. The blood-soaked lash could transmit disease; it also left a man with a sore back for two or three weeks, which aroused "a bad spirit in him." In either case, it reduced a man's productivity.

Although semi-retired at the time of the investigation, Weyler undoubtedly still exerted a powerful influence on the administration of his hand-picked successor, Warden Leonard. This remaining power ended with his final resignation. And although the commission failed to turn up a "gigantic" case of graft, it had exposed to public view its charges against him of mismanagement and attempts to subvert the investigation. Now without power or prestige, Weyler may well have thought the time had come for him to leave the scene of his former triumph. It could not have been easy for him to give up his retirement home, Crystal Farm, and sever his old political connections in the City of Baltimore. The investigation, headed by a man young enough to be his son, must have been a particularly galling experience.

In later life, O'Dunne claimed the investigation had made the penitentiary "a better place to live in," that it "introduced the newfangled 'prison reform' to the Commonwealth of Maryland."[63] Indeed, that same year penitentiary discipline eased considerably. After inspecting the management of sixteen other prisons in the United States, Warden Leonard (whom the state kept at his post) abolished the lock-step and cropped haircut, and changed the prisoners' clothing from stripes to dark gray. Instead of the dark cell, whipping, and "cuffing up," offenders were disciplined with a bread and water diet, loss of all privileges, and forfeiture of earned "good" time (days off sentence for good behavior). "In extreme cases," the prisoner was locked in his cell and compelled "to stand at the door, without tension, during working hours." Prisoners were now allowed to talk in the dining room "in a low tone," to smoke at certain hours, and to take exercise daily in open air. Parole became available for prisoners in 1914. By 1916 they were classified according to their behavior into three grades and granted corresponding privileges. At this time the board of directors gave credit to Leonard for having introduced "a new dispensation of humane and liberal treatment" of prisoners during the previous four years.[64]

---

[62] *Penal Commission Report*, Exhibit D.

[63] O'Dunne, "Mr. Jurisprudence" [1938], p. 140.

[64] *Board of Directors Report* (1913), pp. 8 and 14; *Board of Directors Report* (1916), pp. 7 and 12; and Robert H. Gault, "The Parole System as a Means of Protection," *Journal of Criminal Law and Criminology*, 5 (1915): 800.

The O'Dunne panel had urged the abolishment of the board of directors and the creation of a central state prison board to oversee all penal institutions, a recommendation in part aimed at preventing future wardens at the penitentiary from dominating the board of directors and acquiring too much power. In the fall of 1916, control of the penitentiary passed from the board of directors to the newly created State Board of Prison Control.[65] Never again could a warden dominate the affairs of the institution as Weyler had done. Maryland had at last joined the nationwide movement for the centralization of prison control at the state level.[66]

The contract system of labor, called by the penal commission "the root of all evils" at the penitentiary, did not disappear but did change for the better. A more liberal policy of managing prisoners working in the shops allowed them to earn more money for themselves. This policy was preferable "to win[ning] applause because of larger apparent returns to the Treasury."[67] In 1916 and 1918 two legislative acts authorized the State Board of Prison Control to eliminate the contract labor system and find other ways of using convict labor, including work on state roads, bridges, and quarries. But difficulties arose. All the contracts had not expired, and some of the contractors insisted on their full quota of convict workers. Moreover, outside work tended to be seasonal, and the number of prisoners required by the State Roads Commission was always uncertain.[68] The contract labor system lingered on at the penitentiary until the onset of the depression in the 1930s, when it was gradually eliminated in Maryland and all other states by the passage of three increasingly restrictive federal statutes.[69]

Though not all of the O'Dunne panel's reforms could be carried out immediately, Weyler's departure had clearly opened the way for a more enlightened penal philosophy at the penitentiary, one that was more in keeping with its magnificent modern buildings and that also allowed Maryland to join the ranks of progressive prison administrations across the nation.

---

[65] *Penal Commission Report,* p. 228, and *Board of Directors Report* (1916), p. 6.

[66] McKelvey, *American Prisons,* pp. 239–40.

[67] *Board of Directors Report* (1916), p. 5.

[68] *Second Annual Report of the State Board of Prison Control* (1917/18), pp. 5–8.

[69] On the Hawes-Cooper Act of 1929 (in effect January 19, 1934), the Ashurst-Sumners Act of 1935, and an act of October 14, 1940, see Barnes and Teeters, *New Horizons in Criminology,* p. 534.

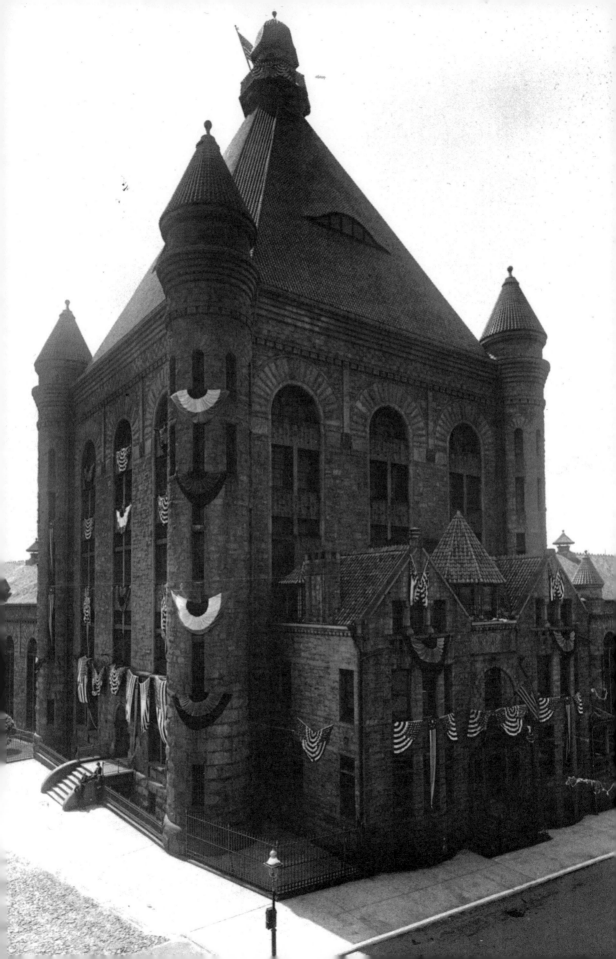

Chapter Five

Reform Methods on Trial

1920 – 1960

The end of Warden John F. Weyler's repressive reign in 1912 allowed his successor, John F. Leonard, to bring about some much needed reforms in managing the Maryland Penitentiary. The limitations of penal reform were revealed immediately after his death in 1920, when prisoners staged a riot to test the new administration. To provide incentives for good behavior, the next permanent warden, Claude B. Sweezey, established a "club" with expanded privileges for model prisoners, an experiment that was soon abused by his charges and resulted in unfavorable newspaper coverage and, ultimately, Sweezey's resignation in 1925.

But at about this time the public began to grow less interested in penitentiary affairs. The reforming zeal of the Progressive Era had dwindled, and the nation was enjoying a postwar economic expansion, the years of so-called Coolidge Prosperity. Sweezey's successor, Patrick J. Brady, ran the prison with a firm yet supposedly fair hand. His tenure proved to be a long and stable one, lasting through the Great Depression and World War II, until 1947. The next warden, Edwin T. Swenson, began his tenure in the conservative climate of anti-communism (the Cold War) and lasted through the Korean War, until 1953. He was more strict than Brady yet professed to be a believer in rehabilitation of inmates. His successor, Vernon L. Pepersack, was far more lenient. He carried on the penological program—introduced at the penitentiary by his predecessor—of treating offenders as mental patients who needed various forms of therapy, and punishment only as necessary. His relatively quiet tenure lasted eleven years, through the Eisenhower Era of economic expansion and political and social conformity, into the early 1960s, when political turmoil in the nation intruded into the life of the penitentiary.

Opposite: Maryland State Penitentiary, administration building, ca. 1918. (Maryland Historical Society.)

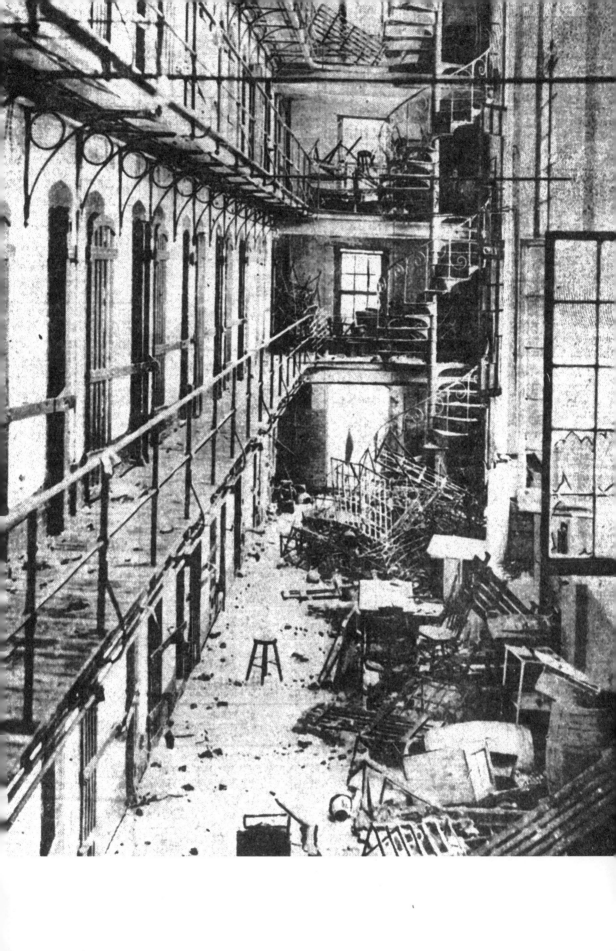

On August 5, 1920, Warden John F. Leonard died after a long illness (Bright's disease) in the warden's residence at age sixty-three. During his eight years in office, his enlightened administration had made him popular with the inmates, who seemed truly to have regretted his passing. "900 Prisoners Mourn for Warden Leonard," read the headline in the *Baltimore Sun* on August 9. A number of them presented a memorial, which said in part: "He took from our bodies the ever reminding stripes of degradation; he cast into the scrap heap the lockstep; he did away with the dehumanizing silence system." He was eulogized as "a reformer with a heart." Assistant Warden Patrick J. Brady was named acting warden.[1]

Brady had scarcely taken over when the worst riot in the penitentiary's history erupted on Friday, August 20. The trouble had begun the previous Monday when seven hundred inmates in the prison shops went on strike over monotonous food. The acting warden broke their will by refusing to feed them at all until they returned to work.[2] Most did so, and the hold-outs were segregated in old C dormitory. On Friday, at 1:30 A.M., fifty-nine of these convicts, mostly long-termers, went on a rampage, ripping heavy metal doors off hinges, breaking furniture, prying bricks from the walls and hurling them through the windows. For five hours they battled guards, city police, and firemen before being subdued. The interior of C dormitory was wrecked. A subsequent investigation revealed that the complaint about monotonous food was a mere pretext for the riot, which was intended to test, haze, or unnerve the new acting warden as well as cover an escape planned by convicted murderer David Bender.[3]

Nor did the penitentiary's troubles end with this riot. Beginning September 13, a series of newspaper articles aired charges of brutality, resulting in the dismissal of three guards, members of a so-called "blackjack squad." Most of the incidents reportedly took place when the last warden's health began to fail in 1918, so that no blame was attached to him for the behavior of his subordinates.[4] And then, on October 12 at 2:30 P.M., the persistent Bender and an accomplice disarmed three guards in the wire and brush shop and began firing

---

[1]"Funeral Rites Held For Warden Leonard," and "Brady Takes Over at Pen," *Baltimore Evening Sun,* August 9, 1920.

[2]"Prisoners' Strike at Pen is Broken," *Baltimore American,* August 19, 1920.

[3]"The Riot In Brief," and "After The Riot," *Baltimore News,* August 20, 1920, and "Intercepted Letter Bares Convicts' Plot to Escape," *Baltimore Star,* August 24, 1920.

[4]"Federal Prisoners May Be Moved From Penitentiary," *Baltimore News,* September 13, 1920; "Prisoners Beaten in Pen, He Admits," *Baltimore Evening Sun,* September 30, 1920; "Blackjacking a Practice at Pen," *Baltimore American,* October 1, 1920; and "Pen 'Blackjack Squad' Dismissed by Probers," *Baltimore Sun,* October 2, 1920.

Opposite: Dormitory "C" after the riot of 1920, where about fifty desperate inmates battled guards and police for hours. The prisoners used their beds as weapons and barricades. (Maryland Division of Corrections Scrapbook.)

wildly in an attempt to stampede the other prisoners into a general riot and breakout. The others refused to join in, and the disturbance ended after only an hour because of the prompt response of a hundred city policemen summoned to the penitentiary. But it was now obvious to everyone, including the State Board of Prison Control, that a permanent successor to the late warden, John F. Leonard, should be found as quickly as possible.[5]

In choosing the penitentiary's next permanent warden, the State Board of Prison Control rejected overtures made by the famous penologist Thomas Mott Osborne[6] and instead on November 8, 1920, chose army colonel Claude B. Sweezey, former commander of the 313th Infantry ("Baltimore's Own" regiment) in France during World War I. The fifty-two-year-old Sweezey, a West Point graduate of 1892, had no theories of prison government but did have practical experience in "dealing" with men, "not handling" them, as he put it. When he addressed the prisoners in the penitentiary auditorium on Thanksgiving Day and promised them a "square deal," they applauded, shouted, whistled, and stamped their feet. His first act as the new warden was to increase the incentive for good behavior by establishing a "club" for model prisoners and giving them a "clubroom," where they could read, talk, play games, and smoke during the hours after work until lights out.[7]

Meanwhile, in response to the charges of brutality at the penitentiary made earlier that fall, the State Board of Prison Control drafted a new set of rules and regulations, superseding those in force since 1889. Among the changes made: abolishment of the whipping post and the right of the warden to authorize up to thirteen lashes. Gone, too, was the old ball and chain. In order to encourage self-respect among the prisoners, the new rules and regulations referred to them throughout as "inmates," not "convicts."[8]

On Monday afternoon, June 27, 1921, the ever-determined David Bender made a third attempt to escape, this time successfully. Having somehow procured a long ladder, he scaled the twenty-four-foot-high wall. Once on top, he removed his coat and unwound from his waist a rope with a hook attached and

---

[5]"Two Wounded by Rioters in Penitentiary," and "Need Permanent Head to End Pen Troubles," *Baltimore Sun,* October 13, 1920.

[6]"Osborne Offer Rejected," *Baltimore Sun,* November 6, 1920.

[7]"Will Quit Army to Take Charge of Prison," *Baltimore Evening Sun,* November 8, 1920, "Sweezey Will Reward Good Conduct at Pen," *Baltimore Sun,* November 26, 1920, and "Sweezey Promises Men a Square Deal," *Baltimore American,* November 26, 1920.

[8]First publicized in the *Baltimore American,* April 14, 1921. The whipping post had not seen regular use since the Weyler administration (1888–1912), and Warden John F. Leonard ended the wearing of stripes by all prisoners in 1914. See Wallace Shugg, "The Rise and Fall of Warden John F. Weyler at the Maryland Penitentiary, 1888–1912," *Maryland Historical Magazine,* 86 (1991): 254 and 264. Apparently, the last prisoner to wear stripes and the ball and chain was David Bender, as punishment for starting the riot of October 12, 1920 (*Baltimore Evening Sun,* October 13, 1920).

let himself down the other side, escaping through Eager Street. An investigation by the State Board of Prison Control resulted in the suspension of one wall guard and two others for laxness. No blame was attached to Warden Sweezey or his new system of privileges at this time.[9]

But nine months later, an attempted escape by six members of the Sweezey Club resulted in unwelcome publicity for the new warden's honor system. On Saturday evening, April 1, 1922, almost six hundred prisoners, each wearing the club button on his lapel, climbed the stairs to the auditorium and clubroom for an hour and a half of recreation and amusement. Six of the club members left through a temporarily unguarded door and climbed the stairs to the prison chapel. There they broke the padlock of a barred window and made their way onto the roof. Using a makeshift rope, one of them tried to lower himself, but the rope broke and he fell thirty-five feet into a ditch, breaking both his arms and lacerating his head and face. Meanwhile, an alarm alerted the guards. Knowing their escape attempt had failed, the other convicts dashed along the ridge of the steeply sloping roof and hid themselves in a ventilator shaft at the far end of the west wing. There a search party discovered them three hours later. Ironically, on this particular evening, Warden Sweezey was in Washington on the trail of his prisoner-chauffeur, a trusty, who had walked off his job to freedom several days earlier. The warden returned to the penitentiary Sunday morning to face an investigation by the State Board of Prison Control.[10]

During the ensuing news coverage, the names of two old adversaries surfaced from out of the penitentiary's past. The chairman of the State Board of Prison Control, Ogle Marbury, blamed the escape plot, as well as the flight of the warden's chauffeur, on none other than the prominent reform-minded lawyer Eugene O'Dunne. Ten years earlier, O'Dunne had conducted an investigation of the penitentiary's administration that resulted in the downfall of Warden John F. Weyler, a strict disciplinarian of the old school. More recently, O'Dunne had repeatedly charged the State Board of Prison Control with failure to eliminate mismanagement and corruption at the House of Correction. O'Dunne's recent charges, said the board's chairman, had created a morale problem throughout the prison system, and these escape-minded prisoners took advantage of it. O'Dunne counterattacked, holding the board responsible, not Sweezey, whom he called "a splendid warden." Former warden John F. Weyler, when asked by reporters for his opinion about the escape attempt, merely observed that such attempts by groups of convicts—and riots such as those of

[9]"Prison Board Finds Three Guards Guilty," *Baltimore Evening Sun*, July 11, 1921.

[10]"Convicts Were Near Freedom," *Baltimore News*, April 3, 1922, and "Board Will Probe Guarding System," *Baltimore Sun*, April 4, 1922.

August and October 1920—were unknown under his regime. Perhaps, he suggested, his strict methods worked better than the lenient new reform policy.[11]

Even the would-be escapees seemed to realize that their actions had jeopardized the warden's new honor system. Three of them testified at the investigation that the Sweezey Club had greatly improved conditions for the prisoners and should not be abolished, and they swore that their escape plot had nothing to do with the privileges granted them. Indeed, they had thought of escape before the new warden established the club. In the end, the prison control board exonerated Sweezey and praised his subordinates for their quick response to the crisis. The Sweezey Club was allowed to continue.[12]

But Eugene O'Dunne's attacks on the prison control board had clearly put the State House on the defensive. In a speech to the Advertising Club at the Emerson Hotel on May 24, 1922, Governor Albert C. Ritchie told his audience that despite O'Dunne's recent criticisms of the prison system, the past year had seen many improvements. Most notable, he said, was the change in the contract system of using prison labor, under which prisoners made goods for outside contractors to be sold in the open market. Henceforth, prison labor would go into making goods for state use only. He announced another important change. Henceforth, all executions, which formerly had been open to the public and carried out in the counties where the crimes were committed, would be conducted in private within the walls of the penitentiary.[13]

The most detailed and perhaps reliable description of the first three years of Sweezey's liberal regime appeared in two articles by former reporter and ex-convict Henry C. Raynor, published by the *Baltimore Sun* on April 20 and 27, 1924. Having served out his time, Raynor would seem to have had little to gain from lying or misrepresenting life inside the penitentiary. Moreover, his account aimed at a balanced or even-handed view ("of course the present administration is not perfect," etc.). He had talked extensively with old-time convicts and guards about former conditions and his stories touched on almost every facet of the penitentiary's administration.

---

[11]"Marbury Lays Pen Trouble to O'Dunne," *Baltimore American,* April 2, 1923; "O'Dunne Replies to Marbury Statement," *Baltimore News,* April 2, 1922; and "Break at Pen Will Be Probed," *Baltimore Sun,* April 3, 1922. The story of O'Dunne's investigation of the penitentiary is told in Shugg, "The Rise and Fall of Warden John F. Weyler."

[12]"Prison Board Gives Sweezey Clean Bill," *Baltimore American,* April 5, 1922.

[13]"Governor Defends Maryland Prisons," *Baltimore American,* May 25, 1922. Complete elimination of the contract labor system did not take place until September 21, 1935, as a result of federal legislation ("Contract Labor in Prisons to End," *Baltimore Sun,* August 28, 1935).

The first execution inside the penitentiary took place on June 8, 1923. Twenty-one-year-old George Shelton, a black from Somerset County, was hanged for the rape of fourteen-year-old Thelma Heughlett (information provided by Watt Espy, Capital Punishment Research Project, in a letter dated April 18, 1988). For a complete list of executions at the penitentiary, see appendix B.

Under the Sweezey regime, according to Raynor, incoming prisoners were allowed to keep their civilian shoes and underwear. Prison food and medical care and chapel services had improved. Movies were shown every Saturday. Brutality by guards was discouraged. Cells were repainted and insect control attempted. A detested, because indiscreet, prison censor was replaced. But the new warden's principal reform was the establishment of the "Sweezey Club," whose members through their good behavior had earned the privilege of congregating in the evening for card games, music, and other simple recreation under supervision, instead of being locked in their dark cells for twelve hours (6 P.M. to 6 A.M.). Raynor tried to correct what he thought was a misapprehension of the club by the public. "Perhaps the name 'club' was unfortunate," he wrote, "that suggested to the people outside all sorts of luxury and indulgence. Had it been termed simply 'recreation hour' or 'first-grade evening privileges,' the public would have thought little of it." He conceded that a few convicts had abused this system of privileges by trying to escape.

Besides adverse public opinion, Raynor mentioned other obstacles to the new warden's liberal management. Old-time guards, some left over from the strict rule of Warden John F. Weyler, would not cooperate, and Sweezey could not fire them. "Politicians" (no details given) were another problem, and some contractors were bent on exploiting the prison workers. Overall, Raynor defended Sweezey's reform policies. "Whatever his human short-comings," Raynor wrote, "Warden Sweezey is a man of intelligence, force and integrity. His administration towers above those of former days as high as Mount Rainier above the Dismal Swamp."

But the Sweezey administration had been plagued by a rash of escapes— twelve in only three and one-half years—culminating in the double escape of notorious bandit "Jack Hart" (James Connelly) and Frank Gilson on January 13, 1924, and then on February 20 the sensational escape of Richard Reese Whittemore, who bludgeoned a guard fatally while making his getaway.[14] This last event resulted in a storm of public criticism and a personal investigation by Governor Ritchie, who called for stricter discipline and the abolishment of the Sweezey Club. Rather than change his policies, Warden Sweezey tendered his resignation on March 9, 1925.[15] He was succeeded by his deputy, Patrick J. Brady, who advocated a "firm but humane" system of handling convicts.[16] Too firm, according to Edward L. Israel, an influential rabbi of the Bolton Street

[14]He was subsequently captured and sentenced to death. His hanging on August 13, 1926, was witnessed by H. L. Mencken. See "On Hanging a Man," in *A Mencken Chrestomathy* (New York: Alfred Knopf, 1949), pp. 121–25.

[15]"Sweezey Resigns as Warden," *Baltimore Sun,* March 10, 1925.

[16]"Sweezey Club and 'Night Life' No Longer Are Found at Pen," *Baltimore Sun,* June 2, 1925.

Temple, who several years later called Brady's policy "hardboiled," used "to off-set the alleged overindulgence of the previous regime," and characterized the warden as a man of "loud voice and heavy hand."[17] Be that as it may, Brady's tenure proved to be a long and exceptionally stable one, lasting twenty-two years, longer than that of any other warden in the penitentiary's history except John F. Weyler.

For the first half dozen years, however, Brady experienced his share of unfavorable or embarrassing publicity. On March 15, 1929, convict Jack Hart escaped from the penitentiary for the second time.[18] And a year after Rabbi Israel's criticism of the penitentiary's administration was publicized (*Baltimore Sun*, November 5–7, 1928), the annual report for 1929 of the National Society of Penal Information described the Maryland Penitentiary as being "in poorer [physical] condition than any other in the East," principally because of its older buildings, cramped yard, and location in the heart of the city, which prevented expansion. The report urged abandonment of the prison and its relocation in Jessup, near the House of Correction.[19] Soon after, a grand jury report admitted to "a little overcrowding," but denied the penal society's charge that the penitentiary was the "worst in the East" and commended Brady's adminstration.[20] Predictably, Rabbi Israel labeled the grand jury report "a whitewash" and called for relocation of the prison and a more progressive administration.[21]

In the midst of this controversy, a botched hanging at the prison also made the newspapers. Shortly after midnight on January 31, 1930, John Jackson, a fifty-five-year-old black convicted of a double murder, was dropped through the trap, but the rope broke. His limp form was quickly placed on a stretcher and carried upon the scaffold where his neck was put into a fresh noose. With Johnson still supported by the stretcher, the trap was sprung again, and he was pronounced dead shortly after.[22]

At the end of March, a new problem arose. The Jones Hollow Ware Co., which had operated a foundry workshop inside the penitentiary with prison labor since 1888, announced its withdrawal to York, Pennsylvania, anticipating that the new Cooper-Hawes law would soon eliminate prison-made goods from interstate commerce. Not only would the penitentiary henceforth lose much of the money that helped defray its expenses, but many inmates would be idled, to the detriment of discipline in the crowded prison.[23]

---

[17]"Pen Probe," *Baltimore Sun*, November 7, 1928.
[18]"Architect, Lock Expert Examine Penitentiary," *Baltimore Evening Sun*, March 19, 1929.
[19]"State Prison Called Worst of Any in East," *Baltimore Sun*, December 24, 1929.
[20]"Grand Jury Lauds Prison Conditions," *Baltimore Sun*, January 11, 1930.
[21]"Rabbi Hits Jury Report on Pen as 'Whitewash,'" *Baltimore Post*, January 15, 1930.
[22]"Slayer Hanged Twice at Pen," *Baltimore News*, January 30, 1930.

The need for additional prison space was again highlighted on September 16, 1930. Nine hardened convicts, who should have been segregated but because of the lack of facilities had been allowed to mingle with the general population, attempted an escape. One of the plotters was Rawlings V. Whittemore, brother of Richard Reese Whittemore, hanged August 13, 1926, for murdering a guard. The other, George Bailey, had tried to escape with Jack Hart in March 1929. None of the other 1,100 prisoners joined in, and the breakout failed, but the event was played up in the newspapers. Whittemore shot one guard in the intestines and liver and left him critically wounded. Guards threw tear gas bombs at the would-be escapees. City police gathered outside the penitentiary to keep away a crowd of several thousand drawn by the excitement. In the end, order was restored, and the warden and his staff were commended for their actions.[24]

A double-dose of unfavorable publicity for the penitentiary appeared only days apart in June 1931. An editorial published on June 3 briefly described the fatal stabbing of convict Frank Allers on May 26 and then the attack on a guard and attempted escape by three convicts on June 1. Such incidents, it went on to say, proved the inadequacy of the penitentiary's facilities and the need to complete the additional prison at Hagerstown as soon as possible.[25]

The other unfavorable item appeared on June 6 and described the recent homosexual rapes of two young (fifteen and eighteen years old) inmates by older, hardened offenders. Without naming his source, the writer of the article repeated allegations of a news cover-up by penitentiary officials and said his own effort to interview assistants in the state's attorney's office had come to nothing.[26]

A year and a half later, on Friday, December 2, 1932, three hundred prisoners went on strike in the penitentiary workshops to protest a wage cut in a new contract between the state and the Standard Overall Company operating on the premises. The strike was a peaceable one, however, with the men simply taking their places after breakfast and refusing to work. The demonstration continued for five days, until the fourteen ringleaders were segregated.[27] In a newspaper interview shortly thereafter, Warden Brady said that his staff was looking out

---

[23]"Penitentiary Faces Jobless Problem," *Baltimore Post,* March 31, 1930, and "News for John [Smith, Taxpayer]," *Baltimore Sun,* March 31, 1930.

[24]"Guard Blocks Scheme of Convicts to Scale Maryland Prison Wall," *Baltimore Sun,* September 17, 1930, and "More Trouble Anticipated at Penitentiary," *Baltimore Sun,* September 18, 1930.

[25]"Unfortunate Incidents,'" *Baltimore Post,* June 3, 1931.

[26]"Sordid Aspects of Pen Life Are Revealed in Strange Assault Case," *Baltimore Afro-American,* June 6, 1931. It seems possible that some kind of prison news management did exist. More than a year later, an apparently short-lived publication called *Brevities* (July 25, 1932) described a near-riot on July 10 in the dining hall by 1,500 inmates over bad meat. The incident did not appear in the daily newspapers, it said, because of the penitentiary's "hush system."

[27]"Pen Strike Leaders Are Segregated," *Baltimore Sun,* December 8, 1932.

for troublemakers and hidden weapons, that twelve of the fourteen ringleaders remained segregated, and that a recent surprise inspection of all cells failed to turn up any weapons. With evident satisfaction he described the penitentiary as now being "a place where nothing happens."[28]

Indeed, compared to the disturbances of the early 1920s, the next decade seems to have been relatively uneventful, judging from the available newspaper clipping books and files. One brief newspaper article in 1932 merely presented miscellaneous facts about inmates at the penitentiary: the youngest was fifteen, the oldest ninety. One Joseph J. Mueller, aged forty-five, had served the most time, having entered the prison when he was twenty-two. Only one female inmate, working as a domestic in the warden's residence adjoining the penitentiary, was registered on the prison's books, the other women having all been sent to the House of Correction "a few years ago" (i.e., about 1927).[29] Two items by a local columnist explained the identity of the human face carved on the left-hand side of the penitentiary's main entrance.[30] Another article noted the decrease in bank deposits of inmates in 1932 compared to the previous year and quoted State Superintendent of Prisons Harold E. Donnell on the chief causes: the drop in prison contract labor in anticipation of the soon-to-take-effect Hawes-Cooper bill prohibiting interstate traffic of prison-made goods; and more earnings sent by inmates to relatives forced out of work by nationwide bad economic conditions.[31]

In fact, the Hawes-Cooper bill, which became effective January 19, 1934,[32] created a major problem for penitentiary officials and made up most of the news stories for the remainder of the decade. Prohibited by Federal law from making goods for interstate commerce, large numbers of inmates—at first five hundred, later as many as thirteen hundred or 80 percent of the prison population—sat around idly in their cells or in the shops. A day school was added to the penitentiary's existing night school by officials, which helped give the men something to do.[33] Inmates also turned increasingly to hobbies like reading,

---

[28]"Nothing Happens at Pen," undated newspaper clipping in vertical file, Maryland Room, Enoch Pratt Free Library, Baltimore.

[29]"Penitentiary Prisoners' Ages Spread Over 75-Year Span," undated newspaper clipping in vertical file, Maryland Room, Enoch Pratt Free Library, Baltimore. Internal evidence points to 1932 as the year of publication for this item.

[30]As the administration building was being completed in the late 1890s, a genial Irishman from the neighborhood named Owen Kelly came by regularly to watch the men work. His face was carved as a joke by a stonecutter on the pier cap of the column on the left-hand side. See two columns by Carroll Dulaney, *Baltimore News-Post*, March 8 and 17, 1937.

[31]"Bank Deposits of Pen Inmates $9,414.27 Less Than in 1932," *Baltimore Sun*, February 2, 1933.

[32]For other restrictive legislation, see "The Passing of the Prison Factory," in H. E. Barnes and Negley K. Teeters, *New Horizons in Criminology* (3rd ed.; Englewood Cliffs, N.J.; Prentice-Hall, Inc., 1959), pp. 533–34.

[33]"School Begun as Curb on Idleness," *Baltimore Sun*, March 10, 1934, and "Penitentiary Population, Mostly Idle, Sets Record," *Baltimore Evening Sun*, January 17, 1936.

music, woodworking, and model building to fill the empty hours.[34] But real relief came only with the outbreak of World War II, when the penitentiary's shops began making brushes, shirts, and furniture for the federal government.[35]

World War II seems to have engendered no disruptive behavior in the prison population of the Maryland Penitentiary. At least there is no evidence of it in the Baltimore newspapers published during the war years. Unlike the later Vietnam War, World War II—the "good war," as Studs Terkel called it in his book of the same title—evoked a nearly unanimous patriotic response in the American people. To what extent penitentiary inmates shared this feeling of patriotism would be difficult to determine a half century later. Self-interest surely played a part in their docile behavior. If they acted up, they might have been seriously disciplined ("Don't you know there's a war on?"). In any case, good behavior would have tended to earn them an early release.

One year after the Japanese bombing of Pearl Harbor on December 7, 1941, a newspaper article quoted Warden Brady's description of inmate behavior in an air-raid blackout drill during which a siren was first sounded and then the whole penitentiary was plunged into darkness. "The men behaved perfectly. There wasn't a sign of disorder, such as yelling or whistling. The men have taken the blackouts seriously." Some of the prisoners were "ready to be drafted," he said, and others "would like to get out of the institution and get into defense industry." After a fashion, they already were doing defense work, the article went on to say, making shirts and cots for the federal government.[36] The law banning the use of prison labor on government contracts had already been suspended on July 9, 1942.[37]

The inmates did seem willing to contribute to the war effort. On February 20, 1943, Eleanor Roosevelt visited the penitentiary's sewing, metal, and woodworking shops and was "greatly impressed" by the sight of hundreds of prisoners "hard at work making shoes, clothing, bunks, furniture, and other equipment for the Army, Navy, and Coast Guard." Helping their country, she believed, benefited them psychologically.[38] Less than a month later, the governor of Maryland signed a prison-labor law allowing selected inmates to work outside the prison walls as orderlies or maintenance men in hospitals, and as farm workers, truck drivers, welders, or riveters.[39] The manpower shortage through-

---

[34]"Prisoners Take Idleness Problem Into Their Own Hands," *Baltimore Evening Sun*, July 28, 1936, and "Convicts Turn to Hobbies When Prison Shops Are Closed," *Baltimore Evening Sun*, December 17, 1936.

[35]"Even the Maryland Pen is getting into War Production," *Baltimore News-Post*, September 25, 1942.

[36]"Warden Finds Prisoners Are Well Behaved During Alerts," *Baltimore Sun*, December 15, 1942.

[37]"Truman Ends Order on Prison-made Goods," *Baltimore Sunday Sun*, June 1, 1947.

[38]"Mrs. Roosevelt Inspects Md. Pen," *Baltimore News-Post*, February 20, 1943. She also toured the cellblocks, and, after glancing into some of the decorated cells on the first tier, was heard to remark, "They're rather homelike, aren't they? You apparently allow the prisoners much in the way of conveniences."

[39]"Trial Due for New Prison Labor Law" and "Prisoners May Aid with War Work," *Baltimore Sun*, March 17 and 19, 1943.

Right: No draft worries for this prisoner, but with only a larceny conviction, a non-violent crime, he could have helped the war effort by working outside the prison walls as an orderly or maintenance man in a hospital or as a farm worker, truck driver, welder, or riveter.

Below: Male chapel in the administration building.

Opposite: Short-timers or parolees from the past. (Maryland Division of Correction.)

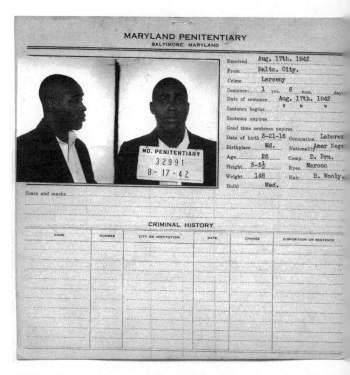

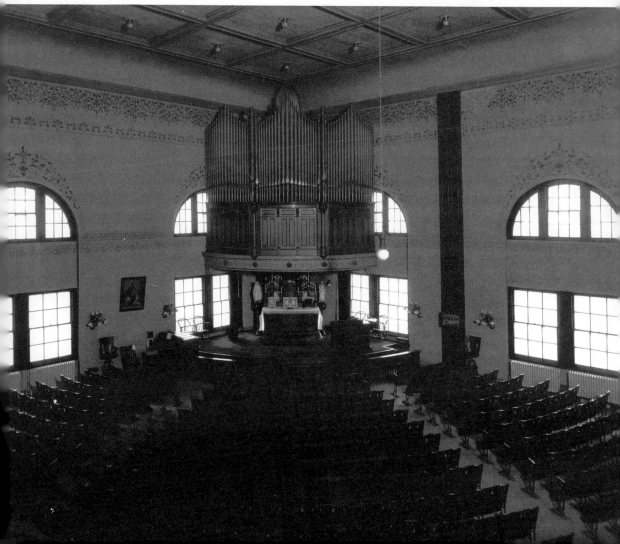

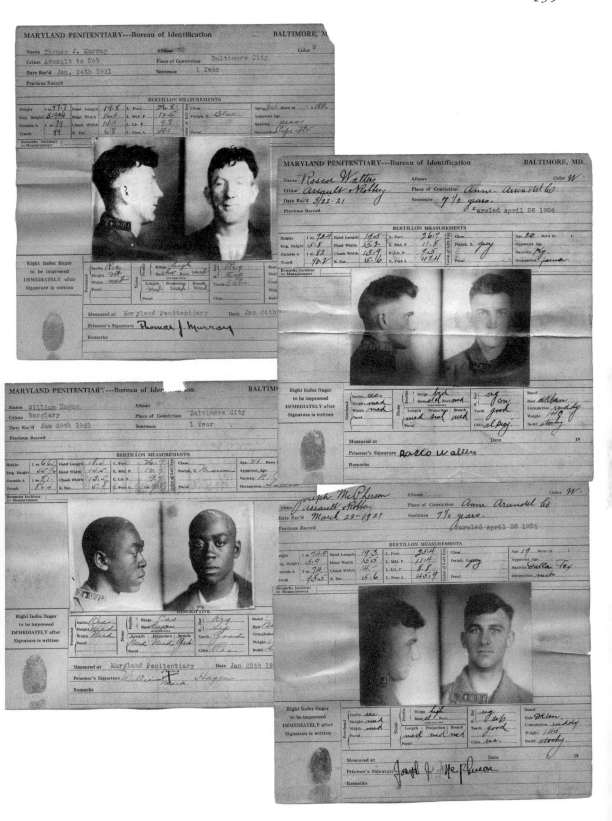

out the country had indeed become acute. On September 16 of the same year, the Maryland Penitentiary shared with three other state penal institutions in the award of the national service pennant by the War Production Board for "labor furnished, material produced, blood donations and other activities related to war needs."[40] Four days later, the state announced its plans to release fifty selected inmates a month into the armed forces.[41]

Not all prisoners were intent on serving their country. On October 26, 1943, inmates Frank Wozniak and Joseph Mahuki used a makeshift rope to go over the Madison Street wall and, having injured themselves in the twenty-foot drop, hitched a ride to freedom from a passing milk wagon driver.[42] Another inmate, nineteen-year-old Paul Black, squeezed his scant frame (102 pounds) into a wooden ammunition box being sent to the armed forces but was discovered.[43] He tried again on June 30, 1944, this time by climbing the west wall with a makeshift rope in company with twenty-one-year-old Salvatore Appittio. His accomplice seized a shotgun from an empty guard tower and fought off guards for half an hour in a battle that drew five hundred spectators along the Fallsway. The siege ended with Appittio's suicide and Black's surrender.[44]

Perhaps the most spectacular escape from the penitentiary during the 1940s occurred when twenty-nine-year-old Peter Bernackie made a broad jump to freedom that Warden Brady described as almost "impossible." On December 13, 1946, Bernackie climbed to the roof of F building near the east wall on Forrest Street. With a running start, he leaped over a horizontal distance of seventeen feet and landed on the top of the wall, an additional fifteen feet below the roof. Once there, he hung on to the railing and dropped twenty-two feet to the sidewalk and escaped in an automobile waiting for him on nearby Greenmount Avenue.[45]

Bernackie was never recaptured. Six months later, thirty-seven-year-old convict James De Michaels tried the same stunt at almost the same spot, hit the inside of the wall, and fell to the ground, severely injured.[46]

The end of World War II meant an end to war work for inmates and an end

---

[40]"WPB Will Honor 4 State Prisons," *Baltimore Sun,* September 17, 1943.

[41]"Services Will Get 50 From State's Prison," *Baltimore News-Post,* September 20, 1943.

[42]"Police Seek Pair Near Hospital," *Baltimore News-Post,* October 26, 1943.

[43]"Convict Tries Escape Inside Wooden Box," *Baltimore Evening Sun,* January 17, 1944.

[44]"Convict Kills Himself When Penitentiary Break Is Foiled," *Baltimore Sun,* July 1, 1944.

[45]"Convict Aided in His Escape, Warden Says," *Baltimore Sun,* December 14, 1946. Further details of this carefully planned escape were provided in 1988 by retired Captain Robert L. Burrell. For weeks Bernackie had trained for the escape by jumping over a row of fifty-gallon drums, adding one at every stage until he could jump the distance. His behavior aroused the curiosity of the guards. The warden even had him examined by a psychiatrist, to see why he was jumping the drums. Shaking his head in admiration, Captain Burrell added, "You generally don't see this kind of commitment in convicts." Interview with Robert L. Burrell, August 1, 1988.

[46]"Escape Leap Falls Short," *Baltimore Sun,* May 29, 1947.

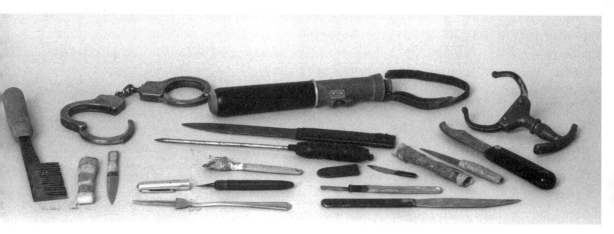

A prison guard's memorabilia include a tear gas billy and an iron claw (used to inflict a painful and controlling grip on an unruly prisoner's wrist), both now obsolete. Among the weapons fashioned by inmates, note the fountain pen with a razor nib, confiscated by Captain Robert L. Burrell when he recalled that the prisoner carrying it could neither read nor write. (Photograph by Alan Scherr. Courtesy Captain Robert L. Burrell.)

to the nationwide labor shortage, as servicemen returned to civilian life. Idleness once more became a major problem for prison officials. In April 1946, as many as 33 percent of prison inmates statewide were reported idle. At the penitentiary, four hundred men sat around in "idle shops," former factory rooms converted to day rooms. The unemployed convicts continually asked for work, which they had come to look upon as a privilege. The Governor's Commission on Prison Labor did its best to find work for them but was hampered by federal law against the interstate transport of prison-made goods and by state law restricting the sale of those goods to state agencies—such items as auto license tags, school lockers, clothing for use in state institutions, furniture for offices

Overleaf: The old and the new penitentiary. This circa 1950 photograph looking northwest toward the City Jail (top) and the Jones Falls shows the original penitentiary buildings (lower left at Madison and Forrest Streets)—the square administration building (1811) flanked by the western (1811) and eastern (1829) dormitories, with C dormitory (1870), shaped like its letter, jammed against the western dormitory. In the middle of the photograph lie the remains of the workshop complex (1836) and the nearly hidden keeper's office (with two sets of bleachers bracketing its entrance) attached to the north and east wings. The west wing has been replaced by a larger shop.

On the corner of Eager and Forrest Streets to the right stands the new penitentiary (1899), the castle-like administration building with the west wing extending along Eager and the shorter south wing along Forrest. The square powerhouse with smokestack stands next to the taller Annapolis building (school and laundry), from which runs the long, low dining hall (seating 1,050), with attached kitchen and bakehouse. (Courtesy, Lt. James Felix.)

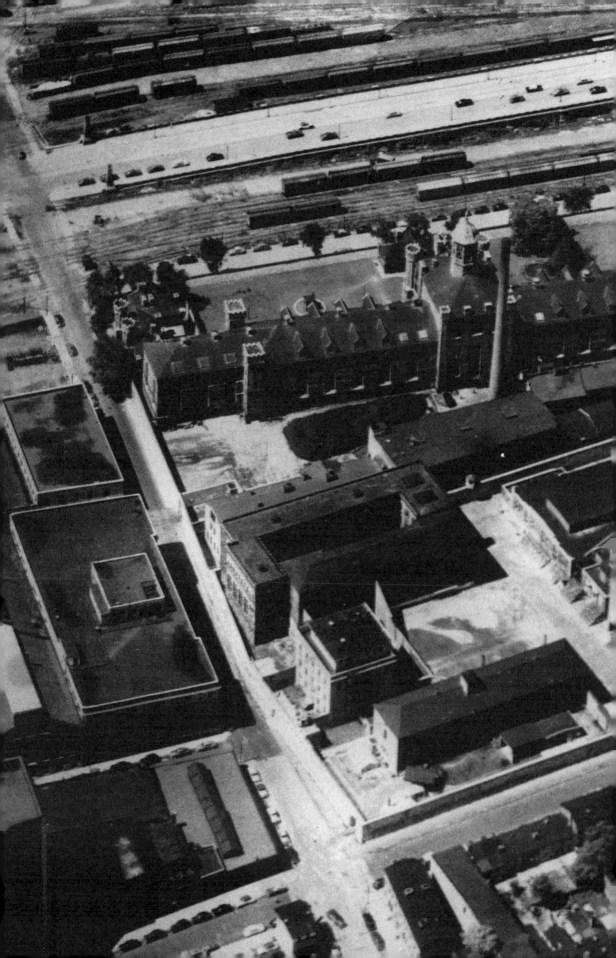

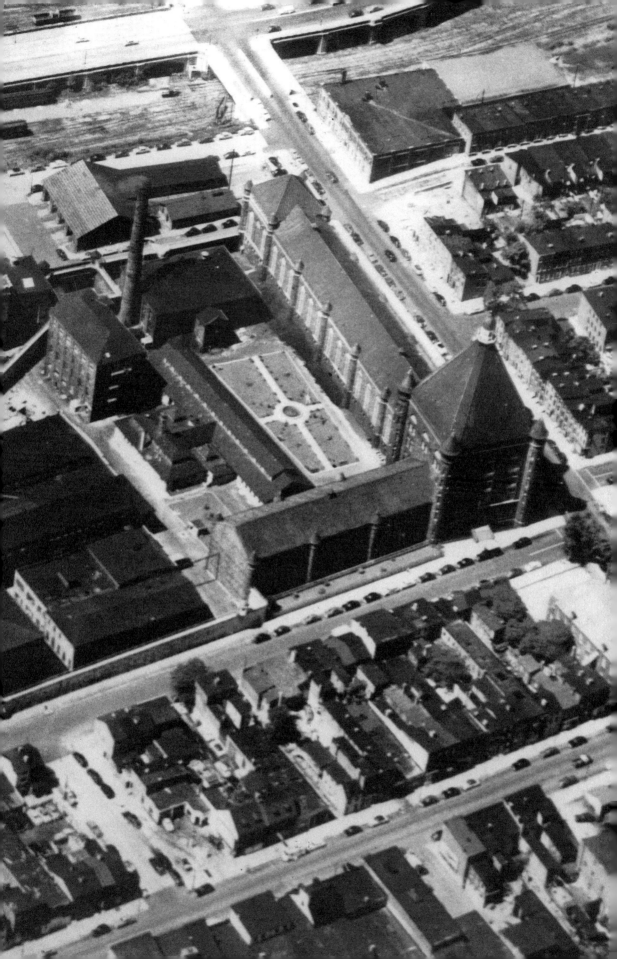

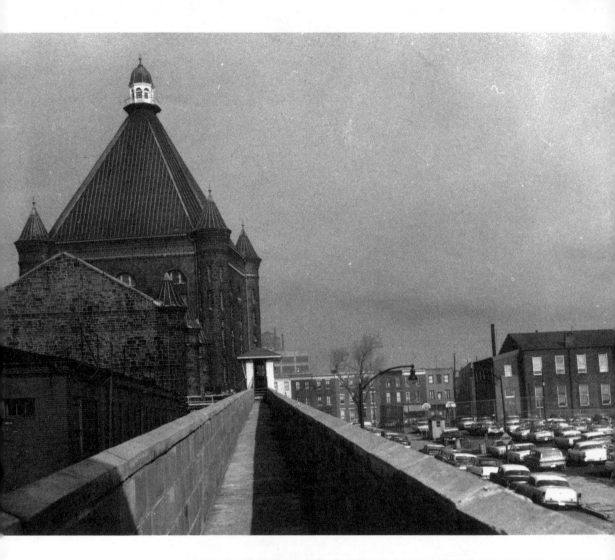

Top: The administration building, south wing, and Wall Post No. 1. Barbed wire was placed on the roof of the brick shop building to the left after inmate Peter Bernackie broadjumped from the roof to the wall and made good his escape on December 13, 1946.

Right: The original administration building served as a hospital until 1954, when it was demolished. The top floor with the caged terrace was used by tuberculosis patients for sunning and fresh air. (Photographs courtesy Maryland State Penitentiary collection and Captain Robert L. Burrell.)

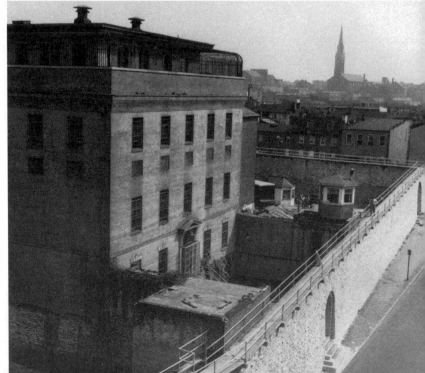

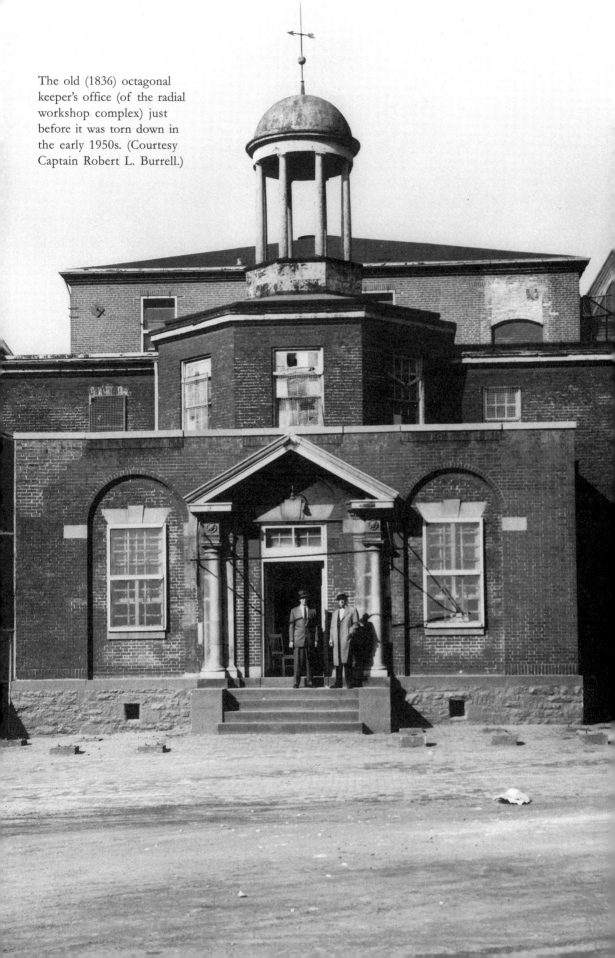

The old (1836) octagonal keeper's office (of the radial workshop complex) just before it was torn down in the early 1950s. (Courtesy Captain Robert L. Burrell.)

and schools, soap, brushes, and brooms.[47] Unemployment of inmates would prove to be a stubborn problem for the penitentiary in the post-war years.

Unemployment—in or out of prison—tends to make people misbehave, in keeping with the familiar adage, "Idle hands are the devil's workshop." A description of such behavior at the penitentiary emerged in a newspaper's coverage of a murder trial at the time. While defending himself against the charge of fatally stabbing another inmate on May 5, 1946, Floyd Madison told the jury that many prisoners besides himself were carrying knives and could have done the deed. He went on to say that gambling and drinking existed at the penitentiary as well. Confronted with these allegations, Warden Brady readily admitted that a "certain amount of gambling goes on all the time . . . just like you have it outside," but for cigarettes, not money, which if found on prisoners was confiscated. There is no regular drinking, he said, but the men did "occasionally" make a home brew, "jump steady," from dried prunes and peaches, and yeast stolen from the bakery. And prisoners could make a knife out of a tin can, a piece of scrap metal, even a piece of wood. "I have two wooden knives as sharp as a stiletto in my office. Every time we have a shakedown we pick up a dozen or more of these knives." He concluded by saying these activities were nothing new, but had existed at the penitentiary even before he came there thirty years before.[48] State Superintendent of Prisons Harold E. Donnell stood behind his warden, saying that "all reasonable precautions" were being taken against gambling, drinking, and knife-making, but that such activities existed at other prisons as well and probably would continue.[49]

In a move apparently unconnected with the foregoing newspaper publicity, the sixty-five-year-old Warden Brady resigned on July 1, 1947, after thirty years in the penal system, twenty-two of them as warden, the second longest such tenure at the penitentiary. One newspaper described the outgoing warden as "a stern disciplinarian" who had "always earned the respect of the prisoners by his personal courage." Another tribute stressed his fairness in dealing with inmates, which undoubtedly contributed to his having a long and relatively uneventful reign.[50] Like prison wardens everywhere, Brady surely appreciated the truth of the saying, "No news is good news."

His successor was a forty-four-year-old army lieutenant colonel, Edwin T. Swenson, a native of Minnesota, who had served in that state's prison system

---

[47]"33% of Penal Institutions' Inmates Idle," *Baltimore Sun*, April 27, 1946.

[48]"Pen Drinking and Gambling Are Admitted," *Baltimore Sun*, June 22, 1946.

[49]"Pen Drinking Is 'Held Down,'" *Baltimore Sun*, June 23, 1946.

[50]"Pat Brady to Retire as Warden of Pen," *Baltimore News-Post*, May 30, 1947, and "Brady Retiring as Warden of Penitentiary," *Baltimore Evening Sun*, May 30, 1947.

from 1927 to 1941, at which time he was called to active duty with the National Guard and became a combat veteran. After the war he served as commandant of the huge U.S. Army Disciplinary Barracks at Green Haven, New York.[51] While explaining his views on penology to the press, Swenson said he believed in "firm and just discipline," administered by "a high type of custodial personnel"[52] and that rehabilitation of the prisoner should be the primary goal, "to improve him mentally and physically and to give him some skill which will prepare him for his return [to society]."[53]

Soon after taking office, he appeared before Maryland's Board of Public Works to request emergency improvements at the penitentiary. The new warden did not hesitate to speak his mind, calling the physical condition of the penitentiary an "indictment against the State." Swenson voiced his concern about overcrowding—223 more than the capacity of one thousand—and called the unemployment of five hundred prisoners "ghastly." Eventually, the Board of Public Works did appropriate the then substantial amount of $74,600 for physical improvements at the penitentiary, including the enlargement of its State Use Industries by 20 percent and to provide facilities for vocational and other training.[54] Other changes were announced: the installation of a metal detector at the penitentiary's entrance to prevent the smuggling of weapons, and replacement of the old visitor's room "in the pit" with a larger room on the main floor.[55] On March 21, 1948, Swenson succeeded in bringing in a former subordinate, army lieutenant Loyal B. Calkins, as the penitentiary's first full-time psychologist, to serve the needs of the work and education programs.[56] The new warden was trying to put into practice his belief in rehabilitation. With Swenson's backing, Calkins established the first department of psychology at the penitentiary and started an ambitious three-phase program for the psychological treatment of inmates.[57]

Swenson's five-and-a-half-year tenure coincided with the onset of the Cold War (1947) and the Korean War (1950–53). Like the Second World War, these two conflicts taking place in the world outside the penitentiary's walls had no

---

[51]"Col. Swenson Gets Penitentiary Post," *Baltimore News-Post,* July 17, 1947.

[52]At least one piece of anecdotal evidence indicates that Swenson took seriously the hiring of new guards. Retired Captain Robert L. Burrell said he was hired by Swenson on September 3, 1951, after an interview lasting more than two hours. At that time there were no training academies for prospective correctional officers, so Swenson focused on determining the psychological aptitude of the candidate. "It takes a special kind of person," he told Burrell, "you will be one of two or three guards, unarmed, among as many as five hundred prisoners. If you're afraid, you can't show it." Interview with Robert L. Burrell, August 1, 1988.

[53]"'He Belongs Outside,' Is View of Swenson Toward Prisoner," *Baltimore Sun,* July 18, 1947.

[54]"$74,600 Allotted to Rearrange Penitentiary," *Baltimore Evening Sun,* February 26, 1948.

[55]"Weapon Detector for Penitentiary," *Baltimore Evening Sun,* February 27, 1948.

[56]"Psychologist on Full Time Named to Pen," *Baltimore Evening Sun,* March 21, 1948.

[57]Described at length by him in "Psychology Department," *The Courier* [a bimonthly magazine published by penitentiary inmates], IV, 11 (Jan.–Feb. 1961). Reproduced in Appendix C.

discernible impact on the lives of its inmates. Most of the available newspaper stories about the penitentiary during this period appeared on the back pages and dealt with the usual prison disturbances that wardens everywhere find troubling but inevitable. On May 18, 1950, convict Richard H. Zlotkowski jumped from the roof of a prison building onto the Forrest Street wall, burst into a guard post while the guard was eating lunch, and was shot dead by him.[58] The next day, twenty-eight-year old prisoner Carl Tiller drank a pint of shellac and died in the prison hospital.[59] In December of the same year, condemned inmate Edward Grear committed suicide by slashing his throat with half of a safety razor blade.[60] Sometimes bad news—overcrowding at the penitentiary had reached 30 percent—was followed by good news: prison idleness had been reduced to 6.4 percent.[61]

But the major story—and embarrassment—of Warden Swenson's tenure came on Monday, February 19, 1951, when the Baltimore newspapers headlined the great escape the previous day of convict Joseph Holmes from his ground floor cell (#119) in the west wing.

Everyone found the first reports almost beyond belief. Working alone evenings for an estimated two years, the thirty-nine-year-old Holmes (also known as "The Dinner Time Burglar") began by cutting through two inches of slate flooring. He then drilled through ten inches of concrete base and tunneled his way seventy feet—removing eight or nine tons of earth in the process—under the penitentiary's massive wall and moat, to surface in the grassy plot running alongside Eager Street and separated from it by only a seven-foot high iron fence. Warden Swenson called it "the most fantastic escape I've ever heard of. . . . I've never heard of anyone digging out of a maximum-security prison."[62]

Soon after the escape was discovered, a prison guard of slender build wriggled through the tunnel and found six pieces of scrap iron, about ten inches long and an inch wide, believed to be among the tools Holmes used for digging. Further details only added to the magnitude of his engineering feat. From underneath his cot, the shoulder-wide tunnel (fourteen inches at its narrowest) dropped

---

[58]"'Mutt' of Bandit Pair Killed by Guard in Pen Fight," *Baltimore Evening Sun,* May 18, 1950.

[59]"Drinking Shellac Kills Convict at Pen," *Baltimore News-Post,* May 19, 1950.

[60]"Grear Slashes Throat with Razor Blade in Death Cell," *Baltimore Evening Sun,* December 27, 1950.

[61]"Project Planned at Penitentiary," *Baltimore Sun,* January 27, 1951, and "Prison Idleness," *Baltimore Evening Sun,* February 3, 1951. See also "Big Drop Cited in Unemployment at Prisons," *Baltimore News-Post,* July 5, 1951.

[62]"Convict Tunnels 70 Feet and Escapes from Penitentiary," *Baltimore Sun,* February 19, 1951, and "Convict Digs 70-Foot Tunnel, Escapes Pen," *Baltimore News-Post,* February 19, 1951. He was called the "Dinner Time Burglar" from his habit of entering homes at that hour, when the occupants would presumably be eating and less apt to apprehend him. In fact, he was discovered a number of times and attacked the occupants with a knife in order to escape. Holmes was definitely a dangerous man. The story of his escape is told in greater detail in Wallace Shugg, "The Great Escape of 'Tunnel Joe' Holmes," *Maryland Historical Magazine,* 92 (1997): 481–93.

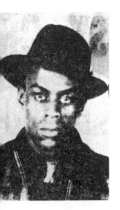 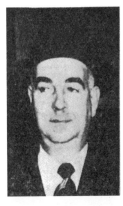 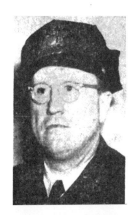 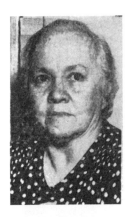

Above: Joseph E. Holmes and three people instrumental in his capture after his sensational 1951 escape. From left: "Tunnel Joe," Sergeant James Downes, Patrolman Frank Plunkett, and Mrs. Mary Ruiz. *Below:* A prison official peers down the tunnel entrance in Holmes's cell; at right another official examines the spot where Holmes emerged near Eager Street. (Photographs courtesy *Baltimore Sun* and Maryland Division of Correction.)

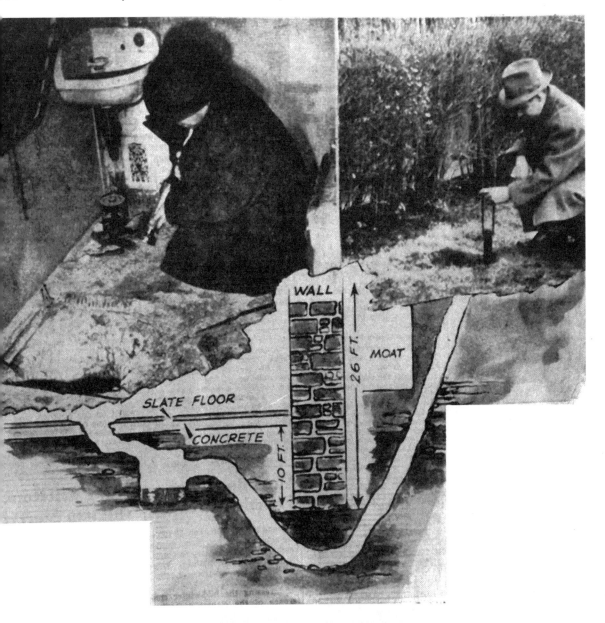

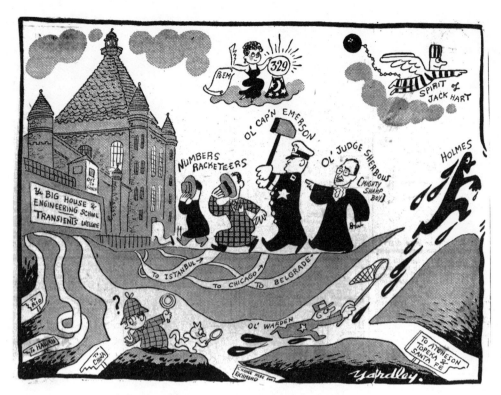

"Tunnel Joe's" escape provided this cartoonist the opportunity to satirize city politics. (*Baltimore Sun,* February 22, 1951. Courtesy, Maryland Division of Correction.)

vertically for five feet and then lower by a series of steps to a subterranean chamber about six feet in diameter, which allowed Holmes to turn around and face forward and dig downward under the five-foot thick wall and adjacent four-foot wide dry moat. The tunnel then turned upward twenty-six feet to the surface. The walls of the chamber and parts of the tunnel had been buttressed with mud-packed clothing scraps to prevent a collapse. The warden speculated that Holmes had probably worked on the tunnel between five and ten at night, when the prison's public address system carried radio programs that would have drowned out sounds in his cell, such as his toilet flushing the dirt away. Especially baffling to the warden was Holmes's ability always to appear neat and clean, despite the dirty nature of his work.[63]

Public reaction to the amazing escape was mixed. Retired judge Eugene O'Dunne, former head of the committee that had investigated the penitentiary thirty-nine years earlier and brought down Warden John F. Weyler, wryly ob-

---

[63]"Convict Tunnels 70 Feet and Escapes from Penitentiary," *Baltimore Sun,* February 19, 1951, and "Convict Digs 70-Foot Tunnel, Escapes Pen," *Baltimore News-Post,* February 19, 1951.

served, "I perceive great possibilities in this man." Others voiced open admiration for Holmes: "The greatest escape since Jean Valjean" . . . "a gold mine of distorted ability" . . . "Entitled to the freedom he, and he alone, achieved for himself." Still others simply wanted him recaptured and locked up for good.[64]

Both Warden Swenson and Superintendent of State Prisons Harold E. Donnell made comments to the press that tended to absolve themselves of blame. The former pointed out the structural defects of the prison: the concrete cell floor should have been much thicker, and the wall should have gone far deeper. The latter blamed the state for not giving the penitentiary the additional guards ("We have long asked for more men") needed for proper supervision of prisoners.[65]

"Tunnel Joe" Holmes—as he was now known to the world—was recaptured two weeks after his escape in a running gun battle with police in the streets of downtown Baltimore.[66] Interrogated about his escape for seventy minutes by officials, Holmes gave additional details that revealed his natural engineering skills, resourcefulness, and perseverance. He had obtained a small power drill to cut through the slate and rebuilt its fuse for the heavy work at hand; he had chiseled through the concrete base with a piece of iron for a hammer, wrapped in cloth to lessen the noise; he had made a kerosene lamp from a small bottle with a cloth wick and set it in a wall niche while he dug. He was not worried about lack of air. "If the light burns, you are all right." He had to dig a drain off the tunnel in which to empty rain water that seeped in, some nights bailing as much as 125 to 140 gallons. Falling rocks and dirt did give him trouble. At long last he was able to make a one-inch opening through grassy turf outside. "I seen stars. That gave me a deal of satisfaction."[67]

He was sustained during his days of freedom by a nest egg of $152, built up from his petty rackets inside the prison: running a numbers game, making book on horses, and making homebrew in the ventilator opening of his cell and then selling it. He blamed Warden Swenson for these illegal activities. In earlier years, he said, Warden Brady had allowed him to earn a little money for himself legitimately "by making things [knicknacks to sell to other prisoners]. . . . when Mr. Swenson came, all this was broke up." Also, the men were no longer allowed to decorate their cells. "In the old days [with Brady as warden], the fellows kept the cells looking pretty nice." With Warden Swenson "driving" them, said Holmes, "many a man goes hysterical and blows his top. . . . I just

---

[64]"Some, Amazed at Escape, Hope Holmes Keeps Freedom," *Baltimore Sun,* February 20, 1951.

[65]"Prison to Seek More Tunnels," *Baltimore News-Post,* February 20, 1951, and "Lack of Checking Cited in Escape," *Baltimore Sun,* February 21, 1951.

[66]"'Tunnel Joe' Is Captured Downtown," *Baltimore Sun,* March 5, 1951.

[67]"Holmes Answers Queries About Prison Escape," *Baltimore Evening Sun,* April 3, 1951.

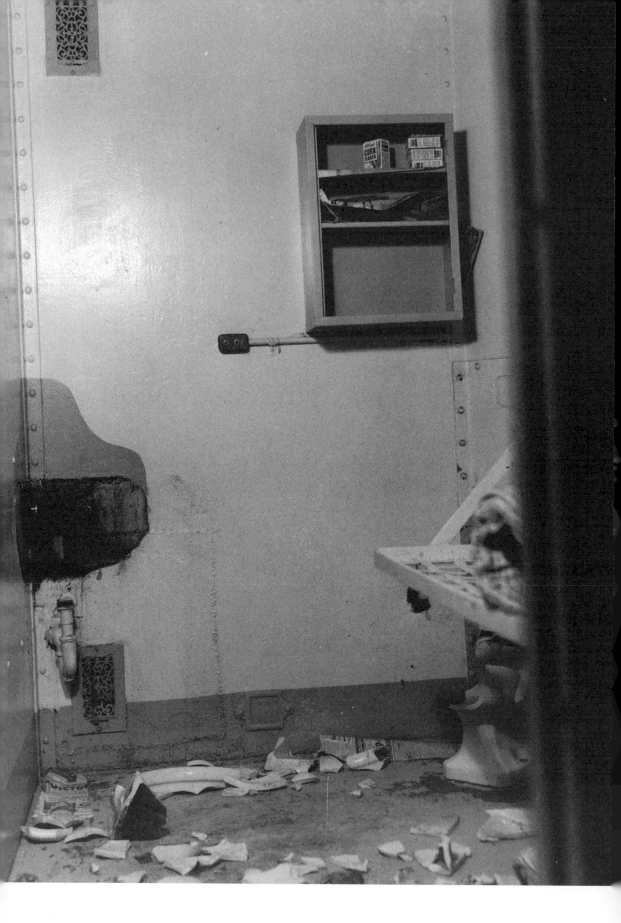

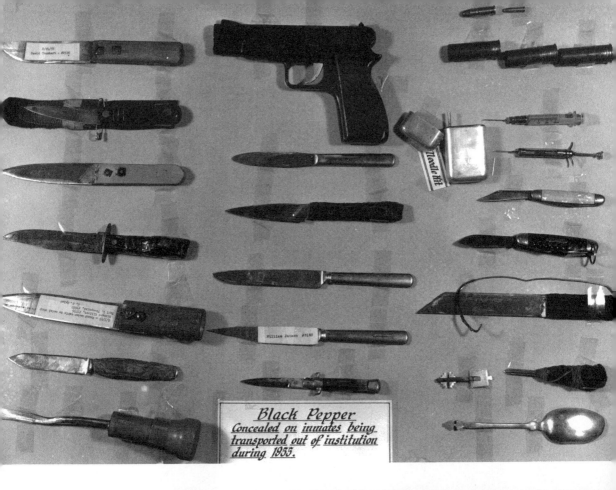

Black Pepper
Concealed on inmates being
transported out of institution
during 1955.

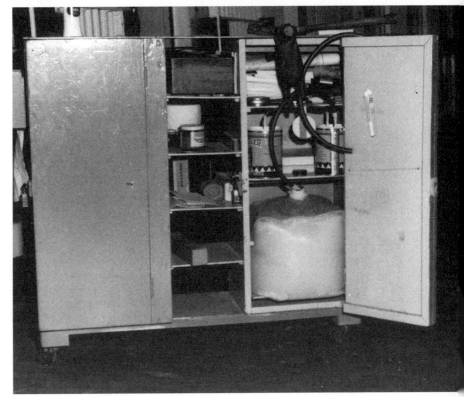

Above: A Colt .45 carved from wood but realistic enough to be used in an escape attempt. Syringes, when filled with dope, helped while away the heavy hours. A spoon handle filed into a key, perhaps to open a padlocked drug cabinet in the dispensary. A handful of black pepper from the dining hall, blown into the face of a guard, could temporarily blind him. *Right:* A fermentation vat for "jump steady." *Opposite:* An example of an inmate's rage is this south wing cell. (Photos by Alan Scherr. Courtesy Capt. Robert L. Burrell.)

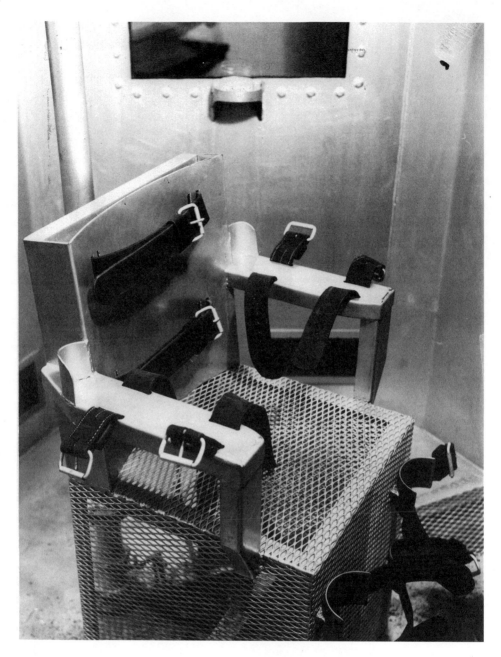

The old gallows chamber (opposite), located in a wing (now demolished) of C dormitory, was the scene of seventy-five hangings from 1923 to 1955. Gazing upward is guard Arthur Wilson, the penitentiary's last hangman. Botched hangings, ending in strangulations in 1949 and 1954 forced a change in 1956 to the more humane gas chamber (above) located, ironically, in the new prison hospital. (Courtesy, Maryland Division of Correction.)

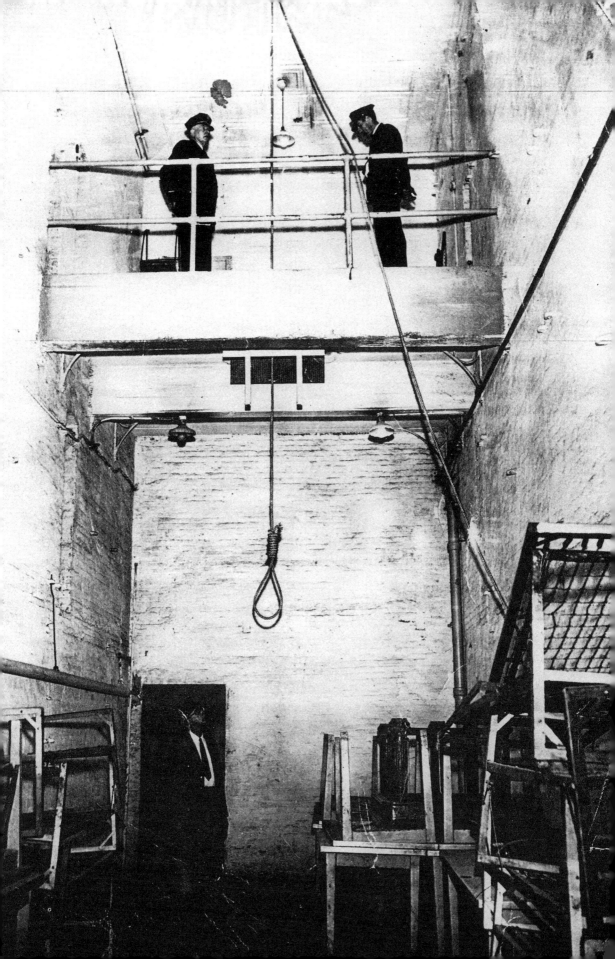

figured that twenty years was too much, and instead of blowing my top, I had the idea to get out."[68]

Other stories suggest that, indeed, Swenson ran a much tighter prison than Brady had. One newspaper article called the penitentiary a "smoldering powder keg," that its south wing had been turned into a punishment section for men to be placed in solitary confinement after hearings by a "Kangaroo Court" for minor offenses.[69] In another story, a Baltimore judge found a prison doctor innocent of sexual misbehavior with two inmates, calling the charges against the doctor a "frameup," done to embarrass Warden Swenson. "They don't like the kind of discipline in the Penitentiary. They don't like abolition of the petty rackets that used to exist."[70]

Yet, conversely, another story suggests that Warden Swenson wished to ease the parole of prisoners to the free world. With his approval, they were allowed for the first time to plead their cases before the parole board, an arrangement described by officials as "a terrific morale builder among the prison population by actually giving the person his 'second' day in court."[71]

Be that as it may, the penitentiary's inmates were probably even happier to hear of Warden Swenson's sudden departure in mid-April 1953 to take charge of the riot-torn prison at Stillwater in his home state of Minnesota. His successor was Deputy Warden Vernon L. Pepersack, forty-four years old. Like Swenson he was a veteran (Marine Corps) of World War II and had many years of practical experience in the prison system. But at the time of his appointment, he was also taking night courses at the Johns Hopkins University in psychology, sociology, criminology, and social psychology, and was a candidate for a bachelor of science degree.[72] This kind of academic background was then relatively unusual for a prison warden and helped make him, as one observer put it, "100% more lenient."[73]

Pepersack seems to have believed in a philosophy that emerged in the prison world during the 1950s, which was reflected then in changing terminology. "Convicts" became "inmates," "penology" was slowly replaced by "corrections," and "guards" were usually referred to as "correctional officers."[74] This philosophy viewed the criminal as a mental patient and the crime as a disease. Accordingly, he needed treatment, which included diagnosis, classification, various

---

[68]Ibid.

[69]"'Macedonian Cry' From Within Prison Walls," *Baltimore Afro-American,* April 17, 1951.

[70]"Doctor Innocent of Prison Sex Charges," *Baltimore Evening Sun,* May 24, 1951.

[71]"Parole Board Hears Prisoners' Cases at 'Pen,'" *Baltimore News-Post,* July 31, 1951.

[72]"Pen's New Acting Warden Is Former Marine," *Baltimore Evening Sun,* April 15, 1953, and "Vernon Pepersack Named as Warden," *Baltimore Sun,* May 8, 1953.

[73]Interview with retired Captain Clarence Davis, October 21, 1989. Davis served at the penitentiary from the spring of 1949 to the spring of 1974.

[74]Barnes and Teeters, *New Horizons in Criminology,* pp. viii, 440.

forms of therapy, punishment as deemed necessary, and prognosis. Though hardly new—this view of the criminal as patient dated back to the early years of the American Prison Association in the 1870s—it was revived in the 1950s.[75] Even the American Prison Association changed its name to the American Correctional Association in October 1954.[76]

Both the words and the actions of the warden were in keeping with this philosophy of treating the prisoner. Early in his tenure, Pepersack set up a system for delivering books from Enoch Pratt Free Library to the inmates.[77] When the educational program at the penitentiary was strengthened with the addition of the first college-level English courses, Pepersack said, "The educational department at the prison . . . is one [part] of a many-sided program designed to rehabilitate the prisoners, including religious instruction, entertainment, recreation, psychological treatment and work."[78]

In August 1954 he set a new penitentiary precedent by bringing in professional wrestlers to entertain the inmates. In September he did it again, this time adding boxers from the Bainbridge Naval Training Base.[79] In a speech before a local business group, Pepersack stressed the need for additional education for inmates and for teaching them job skills so that they could fit back into society again. According to him, job training at the penitentiary took place "in the wood, metal, machine, clothing, sign and knitting shops, plus the printing plant, shoe factory and maintenance department, where prisoners learn painting, plumbing, carpentry, electrical work and communication skills."[80]

A major event occurred in the summer of 1954, resulting in the first real change in the institution's physical appearance in over half a century. The original administration building of the penitentiary—dating from 1811 and converted to the prison hospital nearly a century later—was slated for demolition. One newspaper writer described the 143-year-old structure nostalgically, pointing out the open fireplaces in its basement where food was cooked long ago in large kettles. But now, he said, it had become a "creaky firetrap," long overdue for demolition and would be replaced by a modern hospital (1956) on the same site.[81]

---

[75]Jessica Mitford, *Kind and Usual Punishment: The Prison Business* (New York: Alfred A. Knopf, 1973), pp. 95, 97. See also the extended description of the three-phase treatment program by penitentiary psychologist Loyal B. Calkins in Appendix C.

[76]Vernon Fox, *Violence Behind Bars* (New York: Vantage Books, 1956), p. 72.

[77]"Books and Authors," by James H. Bready, *Baltimore Sun,* October 23, 1955.

[78]"300 at State Pen Going to Schools," *Baltimore Sun,* February 11, 1954, and "Education Behind Bars," *Baltimore News-Post,* April 28, 1955.

[79]"Over 1,000 Prisoners Cheer and Jeer Boxers, Wrestlers," *Baltimore Sun,* September 22, 1954.

[80]"Pen Inmates Learn Skills," *Baltimore Sun,* November 7, 1957.

[81]"Old Pen Building to be Demolished," by Joseph R. Sterne, *Baltimore Sun,* August 31, 1954.

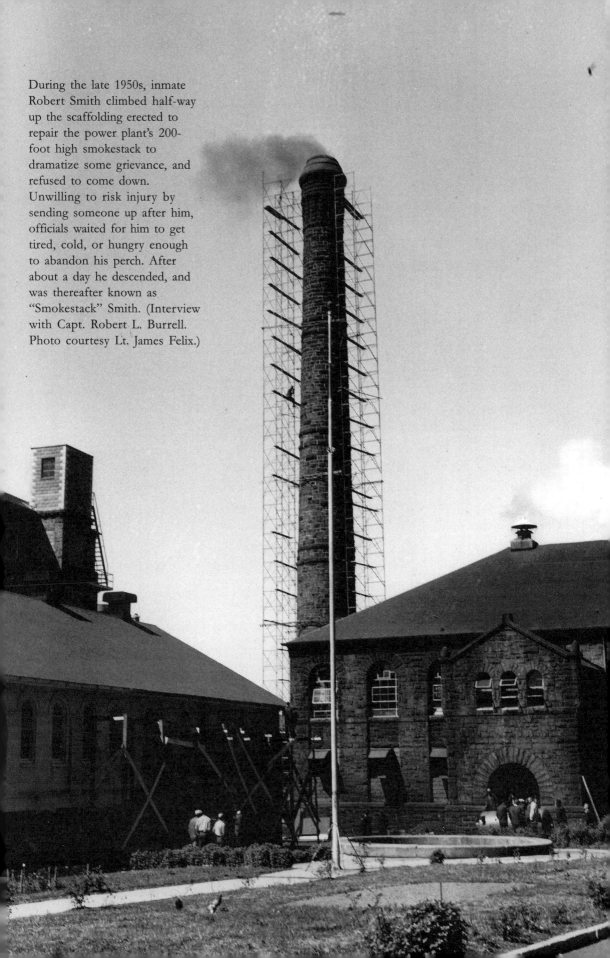

During the late 1950s, inmate Robert Smith climbed half-way up the scaffolding erected to repair the power plant's 200-foot high smokestack to dramatize some grievance, and refused to come down. Unwilling to risk injury by sending someone up after him, officials waited for him to get tired, cold, or hungry enough to abandon his perch. After about a day he descended, and was thereafter known as "Smokestack" Smith. (Interview with Capt. Robert L. Burrell. Photo courtesy Lt. James Felix.)

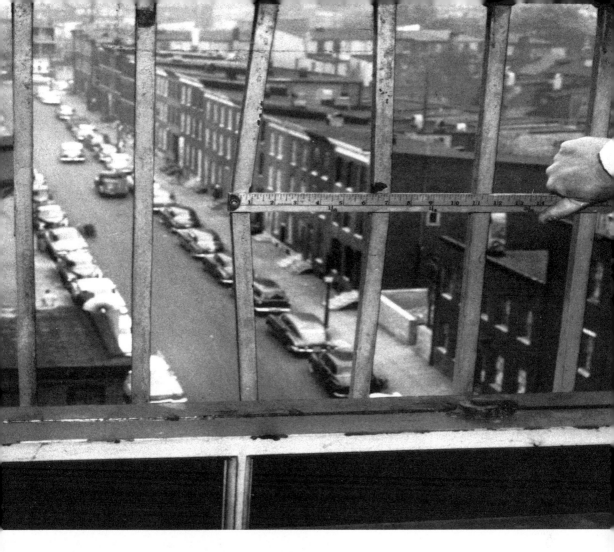

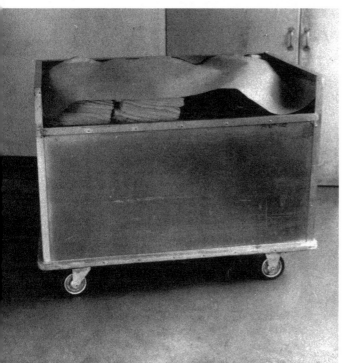

On August 10, 1957, 24-year-old Charles A. Wilson used a bar-spreader to widen these two bars in the penitentiary's west wing from 5 inches to 6.25 inches, wide enough for him to squeeze his slender body through and escape. He was recaptured ten days later, found sitting on rowhouse steps on East Baltimore Street.

On June 28, 1958, 31-year-old Charles J. Yeagley crept under a pile of hospital gowns in a laundry hamper being trucked out to a local hospital. He was recaptured two days later while strolling along Hanover Street near Broening Park. (Photographs courtesy Lt. James Felix.)

The prison routine was also varied, of course, by occasional escapes. On a Saturday morning, August 10, 1957, twenty-four-year-old inmate Charles A. Wilson used a bar-spreader to widen two window bars in the west wing from five inches to six and one-quarter inches, enough for him to squeeze his slender body through. He then hacked a hole in the heavy screen outside the window and was free.[82] He was recaptured ten days later, found sitting on rowhouse steps in the 1900 block of East Baltimore Street.[83] On June 28, 1958, thirty-one-year-old Charles J. Yeagley escaped by hiding himself under a pile of hospital gowns in a laundry hamper being trucked out to a local hospital.[84] He was recaptured two days later while strolling along Hanover Street near Broening Park.[85]

But these were minor news items. Indeed, a newspaper interview with three penitentiary guards at the time stressed the routine and uneventful nature of life inside the walls during this period. "Being a guard at the Maryland Penitentiary is like being father to a host of high-spirited children," said "custodial officer" William B. Decker, "there are no real tough guys — just spirited children, and we don't let them have their way." His brother, Leonard, added, "You have to . . . know how to give an order in the right tone of voice." Most of their workday involved patrolling, locking and unlocking iron gates and doors, and conducting unexpected searches and shakedowns for contraband and "jump steady," the potent homebrew fermented from such ingredients as potatoes, peaches, raisins, and fruit juices. A third guard, Joseph A. Peters, said that only three officers were usually required to handle a cellblock of 814 prisoners: "there is much less misbehavior than people 'on the outside' might think." This remark is reminiscent of Warden Patrick Brady's earlier description of the penitentiary in 1932 as "a place where nothing happens."[86]

Compared to the years ahead, this was a quiet time for the nation, too. Most of Pepersack's eleven-year tenure (1953–64) coincided with the Eisenhower Era (1952–60), a period of social and political conformity. The McCarthy hearings in 1952 had tended to stifle political dissent. The soaring gross national product created a consumer's paradise and a flight to suburbia, along with socially prescribed behavior and dress. Dissatisfaction with the status quo could be found in such books as David Reisman's *The Lonely Crowd* (1954), Sloan Wilson's *The*

---

[82]"7 Convicts to be Quizzed in Jail Break," *Baltimore Sun,* August 13, 1957.
[83]"Query Planned for Ex-Fugitive," *Baltimore Sun,* August 20, 1957.
[84]"Escaped Convict Still at Liberty," *Baltimore Sun,* June 29, 1958.
[85]"Laundry Bin Escapee Apprehended," *Baltimore Sun,* June 30, 1958.
[86]"Manages Children, Some Spoiled, Prison Guard Says," *Baltimore Sun,* January 19, 1958. Leonard Decker would go on to serve briefly as penitentiary warden, from October 13, 1971, to July 31, 1972.

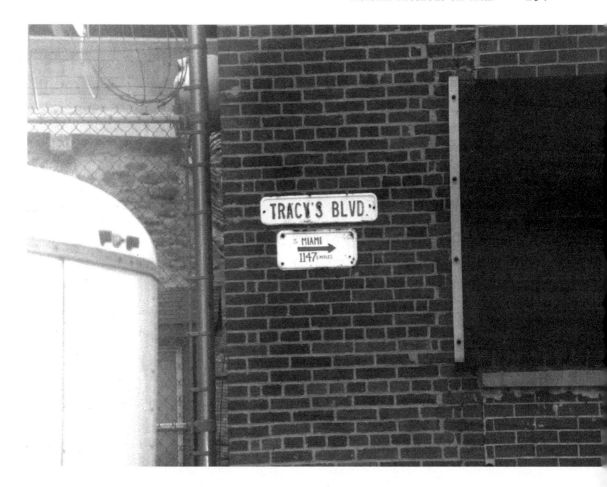

These signs, made in the 1950s by inmates and attached to the wall of the former license & tag shop (originally G dormitory) in yard #4, were allowed to stand by penitentiary officials. The top sign is a tribute to a veteran guard popular with the prisoners. The other is a harmless expression of inmate yearning and points in the right direction. (Photograph by Meredith Britton. Courtesy Andrew Stritch.)

Man in the Gray Flannel Suit (1955), William H. Whyte Jr.'s *The Organization Man* (1956), John Keats's *The Crack in the Picture Window* (1957), and Vance Packard's *The Status Seekers* (1959).[87] But these few scattered voices of dissent were not heard inside the penitentiary. It would take the political mass movements of the 1960s to influence the lives of inmates and their keepers.

---

[87]David Farber, *The Age of Great Dreams: America in the 1960s* (New York: Hill & Wang, 1994), pp. 8, 9, 23, 242.

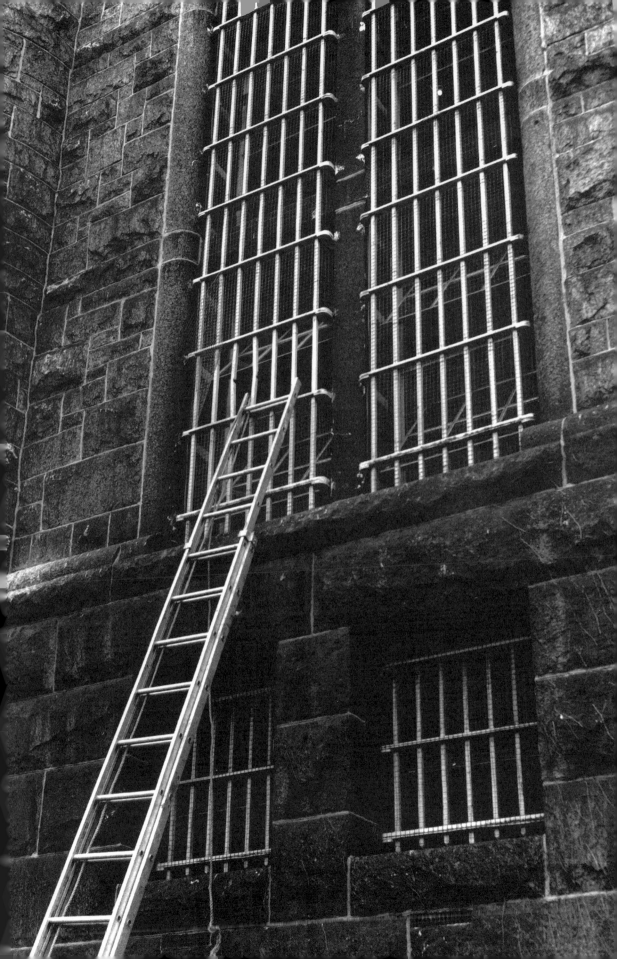

Chapter Six

The Years of Political Turmoil

1960 – 1980

T he two largest mass political movements of the 1960s were for civil rights and against the war in Vietnam. The first, principally the struggle of blacks for social, economic, and political justice, began to achieve militancy in the 1950s and entered a climactic phase in 1963 with the protest marches in Birmingham, Alabama, and the jailing of Martin Luther King Jr., then continued to make news thereafter in sporadic demonstrations or riots. The second, anti-war sentiment, began in August 1964 after reported attacks by North Vietnamese torpedo boats on American destroyers in the Gulf of Tonkin and retaliatory air strikes ordered by President Lyndon B. Johnson led to increased American military involvement in Southeast Asia. It reached a climax with massive demonstrations in the fall of 1969 and lost much of its momentum after the 1973 signing of the peace pacts in Paris by representatives of the United States, North and South Vietnam, and the National Liberation Front. Both of these movements, of course, received extensive coverage by the media and so reached the eyes and ears of prisoners across the country.

While national issues politicized inmates, another development ensured there would be more of them. The widespread use of illegal drugs, though not organized or in the strict sense political but certainly epidemic in the latter 1960s, proved exceedingly disruptive. Offenders convicted of drug-related crimes, most of them young, filled the nation's jails and prisons beyond their capacities, raising tensions among prisoners and between them and their keepers.

The Maryland Penitentiary would be affected by this turmoil for better and for worse. On the positive side, the prison inmate population became desegregated and

Opposite: Escape route of Calvin E. Lee, #9711, October 16, 1969. Note cut screen and slightly spread bars. (Courtesy, Captain Robert Lee Burrell.)

blacks were hired in larger numbers as correctional officers to approach more nearly the percentage of black inmates. Prisoners were enabled to seek redress for such wrongs as guard brutality or overcrowded conditions through the State Inmate Grievance Commission or inmate advocacy groups, or even by filing suit in federal court. In the liberal climate of this period, prison officials placed a new emphasis on rehabilitating inmates through education, narcotics treatment, psychological help, community corrections, and job training. On the negative side, inmates assaulted one another and correctional officers more frequently, and more riots or disruptive incidents occurred involving large numbers of organized inmates.

Until the 1960s, the Maryland Penitentiary was racially segregated, as it had been for most of its long history.[1] Photographs taken around 1890 show black and white prisoners in separate lines entering the old mess hall (now housing the sewing and print shops), where presumably they sat at separate tables. Certainly, as the decade of the 1960s began, blacks and whites occupied separate tiers in the dormitories[2] and sat on separate sides of the penitentiary auditorium. But the Civil Rights Movement led by Martin Luther King Jr. was even then making itself felt inside the penitentiary.

The 1962 Christmas issue of the inmate-run magazine, *The Courier*, published a group photo of twenty-one blacks that tells its own story. Most are smiling or wear affable expressions. But three of them, seated front and center, look serious and have raised their clenched fists in the Black Power salute. It was an early sign of awareness in black inmates of the Civil Rights Movement taking place in the world outside the prison walls. This militant spirit may have owed something to a visitor to the penitentiary only six weeks earlier.

On November 17, 1962, comedian and black activist Dick Gregory came to the penitentiary auditorium to give a performance and found whites sitting on one side, blacks on the other. He refused to proceed until the audience integrated itself, which it did for that one show only. The penitentiary was not desegregated then and there, but according to Baltimore black activist Leo Burroughs, there were signs of gradual desegregation throughout the prison system "beginning in 1966, more so by 1968."[3]

---

[1]Before the construction of G dormitory with its 320 single cells in 1829, segregation of blacks and whites would have been somewhat difficult, because the penitentiary's only dormitory had twenty-seven congregate night rooms, each holding seven to ten inmates (see chapter one).

[2]According to an anecdote told by retired Captain Robert L. Burrell: "I was working the night shift in the old C-Dorm in the late 1950s. A black inmate was released from the hospital and returned to me to be put in a cell. All the cells on the black tiers were filled, but there was space in the third tier, which was all-white. I called the night shift captain and asked if I could put the black inmate in an empty cell on the white tier. He answered, 'No way—there would be a riot.'" Interview with Robert L. Burrell, August 16, 1989.

[3]Interview with Leo Burroughs Jr. (October 1, 1989), who as an official of the Congress of Racial Equality and the local integrationist Civic Interest Group was a leader of protests against segregation in Maryland's

In April 1963 a climactic phase of the Civil Rights Movement occurred when Martin Luther King was jailed in Birmingham, Alabama, for leading protest marches against segregation. The ensuing dramatic confrontation between marchers and police—who used fire hoses, clubs, and dogs against black women and children—was played up in the newspapers and on television and would certainly have fueled the discontent of black inmates throughout the Maryland prison system.

Along with the ongoing Civil Rights Movement in 1963 came a decision from the Supreme Court that would help engender a new spirit of militance in prisoners at the penitentiary, black and white alike. After five years spent on the penitentiary's death row, convicted killer John Leo Brady won a reprieve. The Supreme Court ruled that Brady's civil rights had been violated, that the State of Maryland had suppressed evidence favorable to him at his trial in 1958 and was in violation of due process. The *Brady* decision, according to his biographer, "became the crux of appeals by convicts in prisons around the country," not just at the Maryland Penitentiary. A number of similar decisions in the 1960s— *Mapp* (1961), *Escobedo* (1964), *Miranda* (1966)—would in time make prisoners across the nation increasingly aware of their rights. Many would become "jailhouse lawyers" who worked in their cells on their cases in hopes of winning their freedom or obtaining redress for such wrongs as overcrowded conditions or guard brutality.[4]

Like the Civil Rights Movement, the various protests by students in the 1960s received wide coverage in the newspapers and on television and undoubtedly contributed to the unrest among prisoners across the nation, though exactly to what extent would be difficult to determine. The manifesto issued by the Students for a Democratic Society in the spring of 1962, known as the Port Huron (Michigan) Statement probably would have gone unnoticed by most inmates. But the Free Speech Movement at the University of California at Berkeley in 1964—Mario Savio addressed thousands of students on December 2— was a conspicuous event in the media.[5] So were the clashes that took place between police and students, the latter mainly offspring of white, middle-class parents. Seeing or reading about these events, a prisoner might well have asked himself, if these spoiled kids can act up, why can't I? The massive demonstrations by students (mostly white) against the Vietnam War later in the decade would have been even more unsettling. As explained by criminologist Donald

---

prison facilities. See "Prayers Protest Jail Segregation," *Baltimore Sun,* April 16, 1963, and "19 Are Arrested at Gwynn Oak," *Baltimore Sunday Sun,* May 19, 1963.

[4]Richard Hammer, *Between Life and Death* (New York: Macmillan Co., 1969), pp. 279, 282, 285.

[5]David Farber, *The Age of Great Dreams: America in the 1960s* (New York: Hill and Wang, 1994), pp. 191, 196.

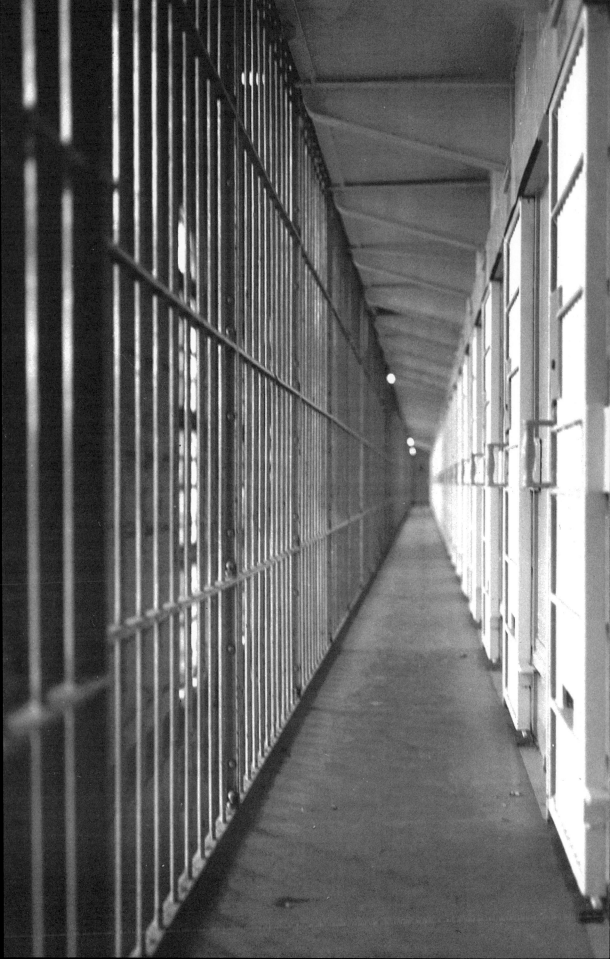

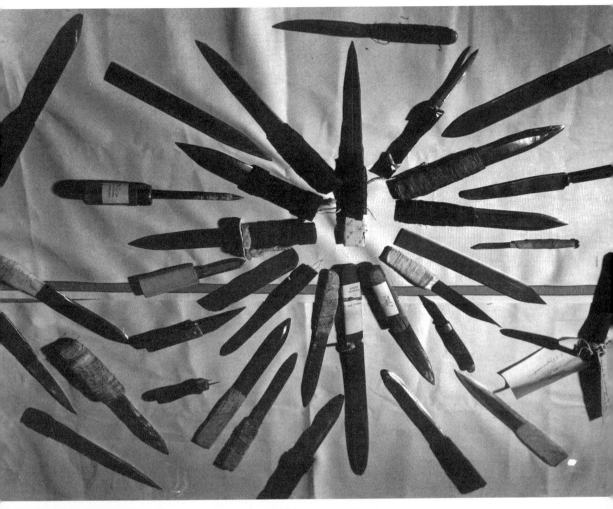

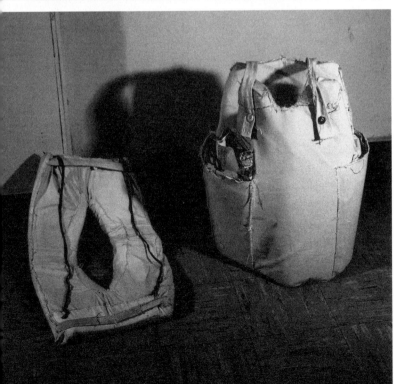

Above: Contraband "shanks," January 18, 1963. *Left:* Chest and shoulder padding made from newspaper and slick magazines, January 25, 1965. It was probably made to protect the inmate in a grudge fight rather than for an escape attempt. (Photographs by Alan Scherr. Courtesy, Captain Robert L. Burrell.)

Opposite page: A tier walkway. Cell doors are on the right. (Courtesy, Maryland Division of Correction.)

Cressey, since "the prison . . . is a microcosm of the society in which it sits, militancy on the outside is bound to be reflected on the inside."[6]

In prisons across the country during the decade of the 1960s, relations between inmates and their keepers steadily worsened as the inmates became politicized. Prior to the mid-1960s, there were enough "sensible" prisoners—those who just wanted to do their time quietly—to balance the more violent. By the late 1960s, according to Jessica Mitford, "a state of war between keepers and kept" developed. Black prisoners were "beginning to look upon the whole criminal justice system, with the penitentiary at the end of it, as an instrument of class and race oppression." They acquired new militancy from the works of Che Guevara, Franz Fanon, Mao, and such books as *Soledad Brother, The Autobiography of Malcom X,* and *Soul on Ice.* Whether black or white, these newly politicized prisoners tended to look upon themselves, not as deviants, but as "political" prisoners.[7]

At the Maryland Penitentiary, too, the 1960s were pivotal for the relations between inmates and their jailers, though opinions differ about the causes of change. Before then, according to retired captain Robert L. Burrell, inmate assaults on guards were relatively uncommon. Both guards and convicts had a kind of respect for each other or followed a mutually recognized code of behavior. But by the late 1960s, he said, the drug culture had taken hold, at first on the streets and then inside the penitentiary, generating unrest and loss of restraint on the part of younger inmates.[8] Retired major Martin L. Groves blamed the changing political climate—chiefly, the Civil Rights Movement and certain decisions of the Supreme Court (*Escobedo, Miranda*) and the media coverage of protests and demonstrations—for stirring up the inmates.[9] Retired captain Harry Loftice put part of the blame on the leniency of the state's prison administrators: "The prisoners took advantage, tried to see how much they could get away with."[10]

Indeed, a not-so-benign neglect seems to have allowed corruption to permeate the entire prison system. From 1953 to 1964 the penitentiary had been run by Vernon L. Pepersack, a man described as "100% more lenient" than his predecessor, Edwin T. Swenson.[11] Pepersack's paternal or intimate style of manag-

---

[6]Quoted by Larry E. Sullivan, *The Prison Reform Movement: Forlorn Hope* (Boston: Twayne Publishers, 1990), p. 88.

[7]Jessica Mitford, *Kind and Usual Punishment: The Prison Business* (New York: Alfred A. Knopf, 1973), epigraph to chapter 13, "Prison Protest," pp. 228, 232; and Sullivan, *Prison Reform Movement,* p. 88.

[8]Interview August 1, 1988. About 1963, an inmate took Burrell by surprise with a blow to the back of his neck. Eventually the vertebrae in his neck became fused, interfering with head movement.

[9]Interview December 28, 1992.

[10]Interview March 1, 1995.

[11]Interview with retired Captain Clarence Davis, October 21, 1989. His career at the penitentiary (1949–74) spanned the tenures of both wardens.

ing the prisoners may have helped allay their normal discontent with prison life as long as he was on the scene. But when, on April 21, 1964, he was elevated to the post of commissioner of corrections, according to his critics "he began to ignore the inmates or to make promises he could not fulfill."[12]

As commissioner of corrections, Pepersack's leniency could influence if not set the operational tone for the whole prison system, as newspapers occasionally noted. In the summer of 1964 he asked penitentiary inmate Donald Warrington, a skilled cabinet-maker, to construct a large-scale model of the frigate *Constellation*. Both Warrington and another inmate, a photographer, were allowed visits—accompanied by a guard—to the *Constellation* at its Pier 4 berth in Baltimore harbor.[13] Similarly, in the summer of 1965, an inmate quartet called the "Wayward Sons" made penitentiary history when Warden Franklin K. Brough permitted them to cut a commercial record at a Baltimore recording studio under armed guard.[14] While these brief excursions may seem justifiable—the visits to the *Constellation* to verify details and the visit to the recording studio as rehabilitation through music—others seem less so, as when a guard captain took one inmate to a local pig roast.[15] Rumors of bribery and favoritism and other illegal dealings with penitentiary inmates would eventually result in a state police criminal investigation of the whole penal system and the purging of those held responsible, from Commissioner Pepersack on down.[16]

Pepersack's troubles began only six months after he took over the prison system. The first major riot of the 1960s erupted on October 23, 1964, at a sister institution of the penitentiary, the medium-security House of Correction in Jessup. The disturbance started after a rumor spread of guard brutality against an inmate who had earlier been involved in a dining room altercation. Rioting prisoners took control of a tier of cells for two hours and held twelve guards hostage. State police subdued the rioters using fire hoses but no gas or shotguns. The supposedly beaten prisoner was then paraded—unharmed—before the other inmates. It was the first riot there in nineteen years. Three days later five hundred inmates staged a sit-down strike in the same prison's workshops and demanded the dismissal of the guard involved in the alleged brutality.[17] A similar

---

[12]"Warden Gets State Post," *Baltimore Sun,* April 21, 1964, and "Pepersack Ends 30-Year Service," *Baltimore Sun,* March 1, 1967.

[13]"Pen Inmate Completing Constellation Model," *Baltimore Evening Sun,* December 17, 1964.

[14]"A 'Wayward Son's' Tale," *Baltimore Evening Sun,* October 22, 1965.

[15]Interview with retired Captain Clarence Davis, October 21, 1989.

[16]"Report on Pen Probe Withheld by Officials," *Baltimore Evening Sun,* May 4, 1966; "Agnew Expected to Detail Prison System Investigation," *Baltimore Sun,* February 22, 1968; and "Pepersack Tags Report on Prisons 'Political,'" *Baltimore Sun,* February 24, 1968.

[17]"State Police Quell 2-Hour Riot," *Baltimore Sun,* October 23, 1964; and "500 Jessup Prisoners Protest," *Baltimore Sun,* October 27, 1964.

disturbance occurred at the penitentiary only a year later. On October 19, 1965, seven hundred inmates joined in a nonviolent sit-down strike in the workshops. Their action began with a mimeographed letter written by an inmate calling for the peaceful demonstration. Commissioner Pepersack subsequently put part of the blame on "the contagion of civil disobedience demonstrations throughout the nation."[18]

The House of Correction riot of 1964, in breaking a nineteen-year period of peace in the prison system, possibly helped pave the way for a similar disturbance at the correctional facility at Hagerstown on April 12, 1966, followed by a truly spectacular one at the penitentiary on July 8, 1966. Like the House of Correction riot, the penitentiary's outbreak began after a rumor of guard brutality. On Thursday afternoon, July 7, 1966, twenty-four-year-old inmate John E. ("Liddy") Jones became involved in a punching match with guards escorting him to his cell and in his own words "gave as good as he got" before six of them subdued him. Jones and several guards were treated for minor injuries. Overnight, the rumor spread throughout the prison population that Jones had been severely beaten. The trouble began on Friday at 11:30 in the morning, when six prisoners in the mess hall went on a rampage, which soon spread into the yard among approximately a thousand men. Four buildings were soon set ablaze, including the license-tag and print shop housed in old G dormitory (1829). Smoke and flames rose fifty feet and consumed its upper stories before being put out. Prisoners looted the commissary, then set it afire. Assistant Warden James Jordan tried to rescue an inmate from the burning commissary and then collapsed. His action, according to Warden Roger B. Copinger Jr., provided the "psychological turning point of the riot." The men began to return to their cell blocks and by 2:30 P.M. it was over. Unlike the House of Corrections riot of 1964, there had been no violence against the guards.[19] But the penitentiary had suffered its most serious outbreak and destruction of property since the trashing of C dormitory on August 20, 1920. Fourteen days later, Governor J. Millard Tawes called for a general investigation of the state prison system by a seven-member commission headed by Judge Benjamin Michaelson.[20]

These three riots of the 1960s were followed by two more at Jessup, one at the Maryland Correctional Institute for Women in November 1966 and another

---

[18]"Nonviolent Strike Ends at State Pen," *Baltimore News-American,* October 20, 1965.

[19]"Police, Firemen Quell Riot of 1,000 State Pen Inmates," *Baltimore Sun,* July 9, 1966. Indeed, prisoners and guards met in at least one place on a friendly basis. Because of the hot weather, a cauldron in the mess hall had been filled by the inmates with ice and lime drink. Both sides visited it during the riot, on a kind of neutral ground, and would greet each other with, "How ya doin'?" Interview with retired Captain Walter Farrier, December 6, 1989.

[20]"Sweeping Changes in State Penal System Proposed," *Baltimore Sun,* March 14, 1967.

at the House of Correction in January 1967. In between the riots came rumors and reports of neglect, incompetence, and corruption in the prison system, beginning with the penitentiary. In December 1965 it was reported that penitentiary inmates were obtaining weekend leaves by paying money. A probe conducted by state police resulted in the demotion of Warden Franklin K. Brough to captain and his transfer to the House of Correction, as well as the dismissal of Assistant Warden Herbert W. Powell, Captain Joseph S. Alvey Jr., and two guards. Other stories surfaced, according to a newspaper account, about "favoritism in selecting inmates for the work-release program, and suggestions of payoffs; of heavy narcotics traffic into the prisons, particularly the House of Correction; rampant homosexual activity that was condoned, poor medical care and favoritism for certain inmates in other areas."[21] Early in 1966, Attorney General Francis Burch launched a full-scale investigation into the entire prison system, which resulted in the dismissal of Commissioner Pepersack on February 28, 1967. Although no criminal charges were filed against him, he was held partially responsible for "serious administrative deficiencies."[22]

It is difficult to assess Pepersack as a prison administrator because the available evidence is scanty and somewhat contradictory. Perhaps the best term for him is "easy-going," imprecise though it may be. Some of his critics described him as a man "with a ready, quick laugh, and a country boy's charm," one who had "a vocabulary of progressive terms" but "only talked a progressive game. . . . The forward-looking programs he outlined were often lacking in his own system." Political patronage or cronyism apparently characterized his administrative style. His own appointment as commissioner in 1964 reportedly came through the influence of a "confidante" of then-Governor Tawes. As commissioner of corrections, Pepersack "appointed close friends who had come up with him from the ranks to positions of high responsibility. Most of them were the old-school guards, many with little education and little leadership ability." And yet, according to another newspaper article, he appointed former school teacher and army officer Roger B. Copinger Jr. to the wardenship of the penitentiary as "part of a new trend in Maryland to attract men with educational and military backgrounds to prison work."[23]

At about this time, too, significant numbers of blacks were being brought into

---

[21]"Pepersack Ends 30-Year Service," *Baltimore Sun,* March 1, 1967.

[22]"Pepersack Suspended by Agnew," ibid. The report of the state police investigation was not released by the attorney general's office until a year later—see "Agnew Expected to Detail Prison System Investigation," *Baltimore Sun,* February 22, 1968.

[23]"Pepersack Ends 30-Year Service," *Baltimore Sun,* March 1, 1967; and "Former School Teacher Heads Penitentiary," by Nicholas Horrock, no newspaper title or date given, clipping scrapbook on file at Division of Correction Headquarters.

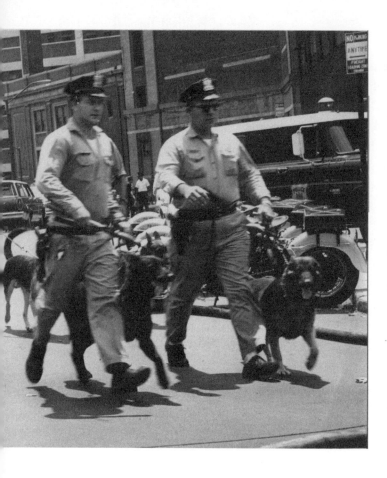

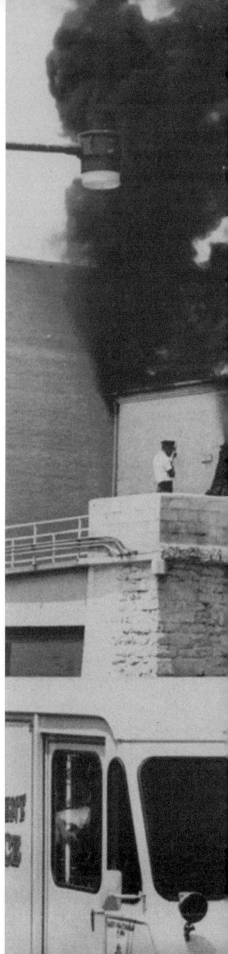

The riot of 1966. During the first serious outbreak
and destruction of property at the penitentiary since
the trashing of C dormitory in 1920, the 137-year-
old east wing was set ablaze in July 1966 and lost its
top two stories (right). The remainder still stands (it
is now the school and library) as the oldest surviving
building of the original penitentiary. (Photographs
from the *Baltimore News-American,* courtesy
University of Maryland, College Park.)

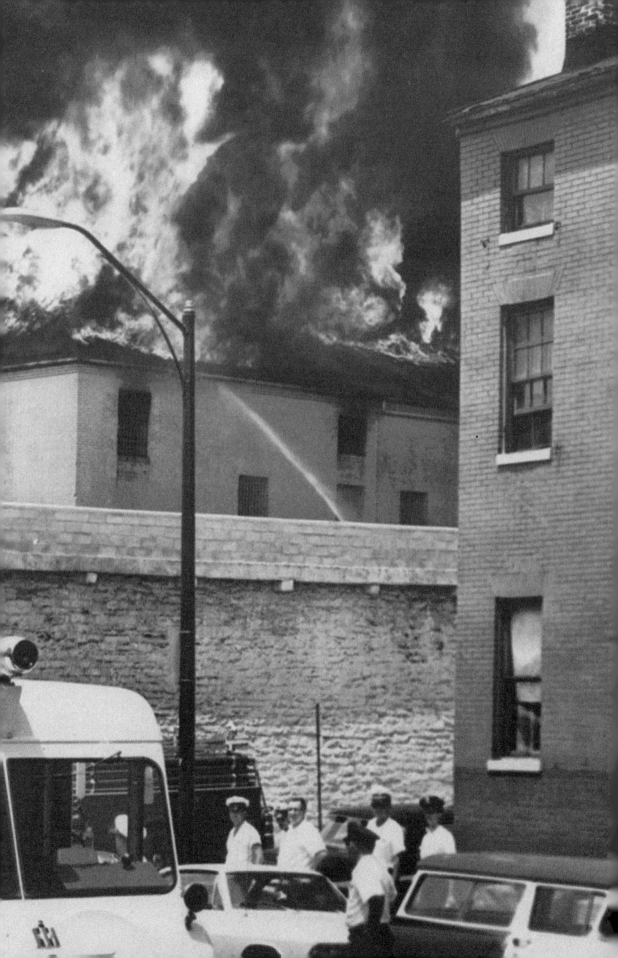

the largely white guard force in an effort to strike more of a balance and to provide equal opportunity for blacks,[24] though it is not clear whether Pepersack had anything to do with initiating this policy. On February 11, 1966, forty-one-year-old James Jordan, a graduate of Morgan State College and educational supervisor at the House of Correction, was named assistant warden in charge of treatment at the penitentiary, the highest post ever held by a black in the prison system.[25]

On March 14, 1967, the full report of the Michaelson Commission was released to the press. It called for a modernization of the state's penal system and presented sixty-five recommendations, among them strengthening the work-release program, which the commission called one of "the most valuable rehabilitation tools the State prisons could offer."[26] The program was intended for inmates nearing the end of their sentence, to help them adjust to working conditions in free society. Work-release inmates were allowed to work at regular jobs outside the prison during the day and return at night. State officials had planned to construct a work-release and pre-release center housing two hundred inmates. In the meantime, the large warden's residence adjoining the penitentiary would be converted into dormitory space for forty work-release inmates. The residence had housed the penitentiary wardens since its construction in 1900, but the new warden, Roger B. Copinger, chose to move his large family away from the prison environment.[27] Another recommendation of the Michaelson Commission was the establishment at the penitentiary of a Reception, Diagnostic, and Classification Center, to evaluate newly committed offenders psychologically and assign them to one of the minimum, medium, or maximum security institutions throughout the state.[28]

Following Pepersack's dismissal a nationwide search was undertaken—as recommended by the Michaelson Commission—by "a national committee of experts" for a new commissioner who could reform the troubled Maryland state prison system. The man who took office on July 10, 1967, was forty-two-year-old Joseph G. Cannon, a former head of the Kentucky prison system, who reportedly had transformed it from something "medieval" into a "model of reform." Cannon told the press he believed in merit, not political patronage, as a basis for hiring and promoting, and that he would use the Michaelson Commission Report as a guideline for his reforms.[29]

Brought in as an outsider and backed by his superiors, Cannon reigned over

[24]Interview with retired Acting Commissioner of Corrections Elmanus Herndon, March 10, 1995.
[25]"Jordan Chosen Deputy Warden," *Baltimore Sun,* February 12, 1966.
[26]"Sweeping Changes in State Penal System Proposed," *Baltimore Sun,* March 14, 1967.
[27]"Warden's Home to Be Inmates,'" *Baltimore Sun,* March 24, 1967.
[28]"Post Is Filled at Penitentiary," *Baltimore Sun,* June 3, 1967.
[29]"Sweeping Changes in State Penal System Proposed," *Baltimore Sun,* March 14, 1967; "Governor Picks

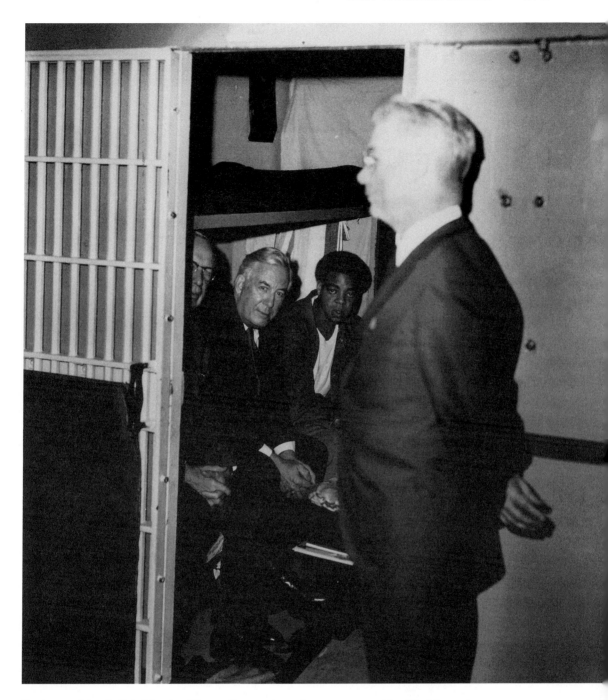

During a visit of Chief Justice Warren Burger (seated next to an unidentified inmate) to the penitentiary's west wing, "Tunnel Joe" Holmes stood among the onlookers and called out, "Who are *you?*"

"Chief Justice Warren Burger," came the reply, "and who are *you?*"

"I'm 'Tunnel Joe' — Everyone knows me!"

(Interview with Pat Fitzberger Gibson, December 14, 1998. Warden Preston L. Fitzberger stands outside cell. Photograph courtesy of Lt. James Felix.)

the prison system for the next four years. According to one newspaper summary of his tenure, he "quickly began pressing for broad changes in the penal institutions, trying to shift from a philosophy of retribution to a new emphasis on rehabilitation. He undertook new programs of education, narcotics treatment, psychological help, job training for inmates, and . . . began seeking greater reliance on community-based programs rather than the traditional methods of institutional confinement.[30]

But unlike the easy-going Pepersack, Commissioner Cannon proved to be a headstrong and abrasive administrator, quick to sack any subordinate who failed to back his liberal policies to the hilt. First to be fired on November 4, 1967, was Deputy Commissioner C. William White, a veteran of nineteen years in the penal system and former acting commissioner following the dismissal of Pepersack. Cannon charged that White lacked the "background" for the job and requested his resignation without consulting the Maryland Advisory Board of Correction, thereby affronting that body. White's forced resignation also evoked protests from his supporters, among them state senator Verda Welcome (Democrat, 4th, Baltimore), who called Cannon a "Frankenstein."[31]

Next came the forced resignation of penitentiary warden Roger B. Copinger on September 23, 1968. Copinger subsequently criticized Cannon for surrounding himself with "yes-men" and being "soft on narcotics and on discipline in the prison system."[32]

Support for Cannon's liberal policies came on September 5, 1969, from a report issued by a volunteer citizens' reform group headed by Joseph Whitehill, a free-lance writer from Chestertown. The report itself stemmed from a week-long conference at St. John's College in Annapolis the previous June. The "St. John's Council," as it came to be known, was attended by over 150 prison and police officials, judges, legislators, private citizens and twenty-one convict "consultants," who were invited to communicate their prison experiences through psychodrama and straight talk, without fear of retribution.[33]

Conversely, Cannon's policies were attacked at this time as being "far too liberal" by state senator George E. Snyder (Democrat, Western Maryland), chairman

---

Pen Commission," *Baltimore Sun,* March 24, 1967; and "Cannon to Shoot Works on Prison System Changes," *Baltimore Sun,* July 11, 1967.

[30]"Cannon Fired from Post as Maryland Prison Chief," *Baltimore Sun,* August 12, 1971.

[31]"White Resigns Post in Prison System at Request of Cannon," *Baltimore Sun,* November 5, 1967.

[32]"Copinger Quits Post as Warden of State Pen," *Baltimore News-American,* September 23, 1968; "Copinger Raps Cannon, Says He Was Fired," *Baltimore News-American,* October 2, 1968; and "Fired Warden Charges Commissioner Blocked Drugs Probe," *Baltimore News-American,* November 18, 1969.

[33]"Cannon Prison Reforms Backed by Task Force," *Baltimore News-American,* September 5, 1969, and "Annapolis Conference Helped Officials Do Something for Better Prisons," *Baltimore News-American,* June 19, 1970.

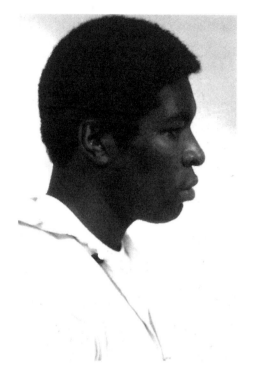

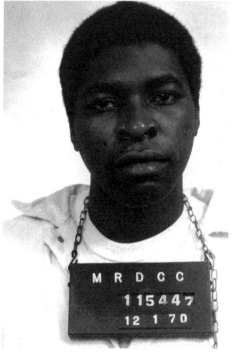

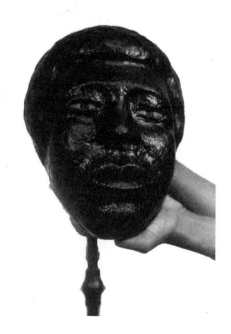

This remarkably lifelike mask of inmate Clarence Butler (#115447) made from wet newspapers and shoe polish, was found in cell 506 of the west wing's B block on January 8, 1971. It was sculpted by Butler's close friend, Harold Waller (#115448) and was intended for an escape attempt. (Photographs courtesy Warden Preston L. Fitzberger.)

of the legislative council's standing committee on correctional administration. Snyder charged Cannon not only with failure to communicate with veteran prison officers and the advisory board on prisons, but with liberalization of prison rules, resulting in increased narcotics traffic and many "unnecessary" escapes.[34]

Many disgruntled old-time prison officers retired silently during Cannon's tenure, but at least one of them made a public statement. On September 15, 1969, the House of Correction's deputy warden, John L. Dettler, a veteran of almost thirty years, chose to retire because he felt that liberal trends in modern penology had made his job of maintaining security increasingly difficult. "Giving too much freedom to the inmates will eventually turn over control of the prisons to the prisoners."[35]

Dettler's parting shot may have sounded like a paranoid exaggeration of the intentions of the reformers, but only seven months later Whitehill, of the St. John's Council, vowed to organize an inmate "parliament" at the penitentiary over the objections of Warden Preston L. Fitzberger. Whitehill urged a penitentiary inmate in a letter to spread the gospel of self-government among his fellows. "You are articulate, fluent, angry and black," he wrote, "will you put those qualities to good purpose, for all your brothers, black and white?" The president of the St. John's Council admitted the idea of inmate self-government had been discussed but denied the council was pursuing it, suggesting that Whitehill's words were "more rhetoric than intent." Nevertheless, the radical notion that prisoners of different races and cultural backgrounds should unite "to determine the direction of their own lives" was taking hold in California prisons at this time and would soon result in insurrection at various prisons across the country.[36]

A second week-long conference was held at St. John's College, beginning on June 24, 1970, attended this time by guards and others who dealt directly with prisoners. One session reportedly turned into a shouting match—complete with four-letter words—between black prisoner-"consultants" and white correctional officers. A media event was staged, in which television cameras followed a newspaper reporter, Charles Balfour, as he became an inmate for a day at the penitentiary to learn "how it feels on the inside."[37]

Meanwhile, opposition to Cannon's liberal policies and administrative style was building among prison officials and conservative legislators. On February

---

[34]"Liberal Prison Policies Endanger System, Legislative Council Told," *Baltimore News-American,* November 6, 1969.

[35]"Modern Concept of Penology Will Lead to Trouble, Retiring Deputy Warden Says," *Baltimore News-American,* September 15, 1969.

[36]"Prison Reformist Vows Pen Inmate 'Parliament,'" *Baltimore News-American,* April 29, 1970; and Sullivan, *The Prison Reform Movement,* p. 100.

[37]"An Inmate for a Day Learns How It Feels on the Inside," *Baltimore Sun,* June 27, 1970.

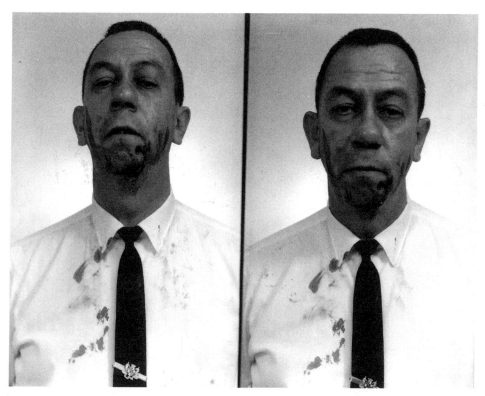

These photographs of Arthur "Buck" Newsome were taken shortly after a scuffle with an inmate in the south wing's segregation unit on January 14, 1971. Twenty years earlier, Newsome had volunteered to make the dangerous exploratory trip through the tunnel made by Joseph Holmes. (Photographs courtesy Warden Preston L. Fitzberger.)

8, 1971, Warden Preston L. Fitzberger resigned his post at the penitentiary reportedly "because he could no longer endure the permissive policies" of Commissioner Cannon. The fifty-eight-year-old Fitzberger had joined the prison system as a guard in 1951 and worked his way up through the ranks to head the Correctional Institute at Hagerstown before coming to the penitentiary in September 1968. He was reputed to treat the inmates fairly but with a firm hand. Along with other correctional officers, he disagreed with Cannon's order for prison personnel to refer to inmates as "clients" and "residents" instead of "prisoners" or "inmates." But he clearly found his job intolerable when Cannon interfered with his running of the penitentiary. Several weeks before his resignation, Fitzberger had turned away three "hippies" from an underground press seeking to interview prisoners. The trio complained to the commissioner, who sat them down and drank coffee with them and then gave them permission to go inside the penitentiary. Fitzberger's resignation came after Cannon overruled his disciplining of troublemakers segregated in the penitentiary's south wing.

The warden's departure dismayed some conservative legislators, who called for Cannon's dismissal.[38]

A few months after Fitzberger's resignation, on May 26, 1971, a suit filed by penitentiary inmate William Bundy against Commissioner Cannon came to a decision in favor of the plaintiff.[39] Bundy had sued for due process to be applied in inmates' hearings held by the penitentiary for such offenses as brewing "jump steady," being drunk, dealing drugs, vandalizing cells, making or possessing a weapon, rape, or assault. Formerly, these hearings tended to be informal, "run by the seat of the pants," as a former hearing officer put it.[40] Henceforth, the penitentiary and other state correctional institutions would be held strictly accountable for following an orderly procedure giving the accused the right to representation and to call witnesses at a formal adjustment hearing.[41] Only since the landmark decision in 1964 by the Supreme Court had the way been opened for a prisoner to sue state officials in federal court.[42] The Bundy case was the forerunner of others to be brought against the penitentiary in the 1970s and 1980s involving such matters as guard brutality and overcrowding.

On August 11, 1971, Commissioner Cannon was fired for "administrative failures," not because of "any dispute over penal philosophy," according to then Governor Marvin Mandel and Robert J. Lally, Secretary of Public Safety and Correctional Services. Lally faulted Cannon for "failures to conform to rules, regulations, and deadlines," including his recent failure to submit his budget proposals for the coming year by the August 1 deadline. Some observers described Cannon as being "casual about administrative niceties, as well as undiplomatic in dealing with other officials." The newspaper account also noted that Cannon had been fired earlier as Kentucky's prison director by the governor for being "insubordinate and uncooperative." Cannon's deputy, James Jordan, was appointed acting commissioner, thereby becoming the first black to head the entire system, which by now had between 70 and 80 percent black inmates. Like Cannon, Jordan held progressive views on penology, but was more realistic and diplomatic in pursuing them.[43]

By the early 1970s, inmates at the penitentiary had clearly become more politicized. In January 1972, inmate Charles Allen complained to the state inmate grievance commission that the penitentiary had refused to allow him to

---

[38]"Warden of Penitentiary Resigns," *Baltimore News-American*, February 9, 1971.

[39]William Bundy *et al.* versus Joseph Cannon *et al.*, United States District Court, District Maryland, 328 Federal Supplement, 165 (1971).

[40]Phone conversation with retired captain Robert L. Burrell, December 20, 1988.

[41]See Division of Correction Form 105-2a (Rev. 9/88).

[42]Sullivan, *The Prison Reform Movement*, p. 92.

[43]"Cannon Fired from Post as Maryland Prison Chief," *Baltimore Sun*, August 12, 1971; "Negro Deputy Prison Chief Had a Tough Background," *Baltimore News-American*, April 22, 1970.

set up a self-help program to teach inmates how to prepare legal writs that could lead to their release. That same month, two inmates filed a suit in the U.S. District Court for $500,000, claiming they had been beaten by guards during a disturbance at the penitentiary a year earlier.[44] At least three typed manifestos from the spring of 1972 survive in Baltimore's Enoch Pratt Free Library from Charles Allen's self-help organization, "The People's Law Society." Crudely written and filled with incoherent legal jargon, the manifestos nevertheless show a growing awareness of the means of legal redress available to inmates.[45] Also surviving at the library is the mimeographed "Dolly Bulletin" from "Man Alive" (a drug rehabilitation organization), which describes—in vivid detail—life in the segregation unit of the penitentiary's south wing. This was dated May 26, 1972, less than two months before the violent riot of July 17, at which inmates displayed the banner "Free All Political Prisoners" and listed conditions in the south wing as one of their grievances.

It was the closest yet to open war. The riot at the Maryland Penitentiary on Monday, July 17, 1972, appears to have been preceded by some unwise actions on the part of the guards themselves. Following a ten-hour disturbance at the House of Correction in Jessup the previous Saturday night, some of the penitentiary guards reportedly "intimidated and harassed" the prisoners that Sunday evening. The instigator of the riot allegedly was thirty-two-year-old Lascell ("Cadillac") Gallop, who was serving six years for assaulting police. At 12:15 P.M. in the penitentiary's kitchen Gallop threw an acid solution in the face of Sergeant William Bevans. A guard lieutenant came from the dining room to intervene but was attacked by six inmates. Gallop stabbed him in the back with a large "shank" or homemade knife.[46]

Outside the kitchen, a dozen inmates ran across the volleyball court to the wood and metal shop at the southwest end and began smashing windows and starting fires that eventually grew to a four-alarm blaze. Attracted by the commotion, other inmates from nearby shops poured into the court, but only a few joined the rioters; the rest took refuge in their cells. The guards on the wall held their fire because no prisoners were trying to escape.

In the #3 yard, inmate Gallop pursued Sergeant Bevans. Gallop threw a six-foot-long iron bar, javelin fashion, that struck Bevans in the back and knocked him to the ground.[47] Soon after, veteran guard Captain Clarence Davis entered

---

[44]"Inmates' Law Class Rejected," *Baltimore News-American,* January 7, 1972; "Inmates Claim Beatings, Sue for $500,000." *Baltimore News-American,* January 13, 1972.

[45]March 20 and April 8, 1972, vertical file, Maryland Room, Enoch Pratt Free Library, Baltimore.

[46]"Convicts Riot at State Pen for Six Hours," *Baltimore Sun,* July 18, 1972; charge sheet on Lascell Gallop (#108-613) on file in the chief of security's office, Maryland Penitentiary.

[47]Charge sheet on Lascell Gallop (#108-613).

the dining hall seeking classification supervisor Charles Gilfuss and Nathan Pashen, assistant superintendent at the prison reception center. When the trio emerged, Gallop and other inmates armed with clubs took them hostage. Twenty-year-old Franklin Henson, serving twenty years for attempted rape, threatened Davis with one half of a pair of tin snips. The inmates then robbed Davis of his wallet, tear gas billy, and handcuffs, which they used to handcuff him to Charles Gilfuss. The hostages were then led beneath the end of the south wing to parley with prison officials. "I didn't resist," Davis recalled, "it wouldn't have done any good—I just ignored them."[48]

When inmate demands were not immediately met, the hostages—now joined by woodshop foreman Peter Myers—were taken inside the four-story Annapolis building that housed schoolrooms, offices, and laundry off the southwest end of the dining hall. There the rioters trashed the offices. "They led us from room to room," Davis said, "they didn't know quite what to do with us."[49]

At one point, Davis and Gilfuss were blindfolded and led onto the fire escape on the fourth story. The rioters threatened to push them over the edge unless Representative Parren J. Mitchell was brought in to take part in the negotiations. Half a block away in the administration building, a young social worker, Alan D. Eason, watched the scene from a window in the chapel on the third floor. "I could see a blindfolded man on the fire escape with an inmate brandishing a club," he recalled, "it seemed unreal, that something horrible might happen, as if all conventions had fallen away."[50]

The rioters threatened to kill the hostages if firemen were allowed in to fight the fires, but Baltimore Police Commissioner Donald G. Pomerleau took a chance and ordered the firemen in anyway. The hostages were spared, but others fared less well during the riot. A woodshop foreman received a head wound requiring several stitches, and three guards were injured, one of them seriously enough to be hospitalized.[51]

Negotiations began in earnest with the arrival of Representative Mitchell at 3 P.M. and Governor Mandel less than an hour later. The inmates presented a list of their grievances. Among other things, they complained about the poor quality of the food and its insufficient quantity, the use of the south wing as a punishment center, and the violation of their rights by the guards. In particular, they wanted Assistant Warden McLindsey Hawkins fired and had earlier dis-

---

[48]Interview with retired captain Clarence Davis, October 21, 1989, and charge sheet on Franklin Henson (#106-286) on file in the Chief of Security's office, Maryland Penitentiary.

[49]Interview with Clarence Davis, October 21, 1989.

[50]"Convicts Riot at State Pen," *Baltimore Sun,* July 18, 1972, and interview with Assistant State's Attorney General Alan D. Eason, November 21, 1989.

[51]"Convicts Riot at State Pen for Six Hours," *Baltimore Sun,* July 18, 1972.

played a sign to that effect, along with another bearing one of the slogans of the day: "Free All Political Prisoners." Outside the walls, about thirty protesters belonging to Youth Against War and Fascism picketed the penitentiary, chanting "we want no reprisals" and "support prisoners' demands." After Governor Mandel promised the rioters that no reprisals—either physical or mental—would be taken, a settlement was reached at 6:15 P.M., over six hours after the riot began.[52]

Many of the guards and other prison personnel, furious at the seemingly lenient terms of the settlement, staged three walkouts in the next four days. After negotiating with the dissidents, state corrections chief Robert J. Lally imposed an indefinite ban on all visitors, including newsmen, attorneys, and any legislators aiming, he said, "to get a little publicity and shoot their mouths off," a covert reference to Representative Parren J. Mitchell, widely regarded as a disruptive influence. A massive shakedown of the penitentiary, lasting several days, turned up dozens of weapons and—in the prison auditorium, where inmate self-help groups had met with visitors—evidence of drug and liquor consumption and "love-ins" held by inmates with their wives and girlfriends on beds and mattresses hidden behind the curtain.[53]

The aftermath of the riot included a backlash of conservative opinion. Delegate Edward J. Dabroski (Democrat, Baltimore, 1st), a member of a committee studying prison conditions, said his visit to the penitentiary three weeks before the riot strengthened his belief that conditions were not so bad as depicted in recent newspaper articles. While walking through the segregation unit he "became totally disheartened and disgusted" by "the do-gooders on my committee with their notebooks out soliciting grievances from these criminals." Rehabilitation programs were being damaged, he said, by "young politicized inmates."[54] A subsequent grand jury report blamed the July riot on unrest created by outside agitators, drug smugglers, and inmate self-help groups involving visitors. It proposed that "the hardened criminal who has not shown any response to rehabilitation should be separated in a compound or stockade under strict armed guard supervision."[55]

Eventually, the normal prison routine was restored, but officials at the penitentiary had learned some lessons that would prove valuable in quelling the

---

[52]Ibid., and "30 Pickets Back Convicts," *Baltimore Sun,* July 18, 1972.

[53]"Pen declared off limits to some officials," *Baltimore News-American,* July 21, 1972; interview with former penitentiary warden Gerald H. McClellan, December 18, 1989; and "Pen Shakedown Reported to Yield Dozens of Weapons," *Baltimore Sun,* July 21, 1972.

[54]"Prisoner Aid Plans Are Rated Failures," *Baltimore News-American,* August 9, 1972.

[55]"Grand Jury Blames Riot at Penitentiary on Outsiders," *Baltimore News-American,* September 10, 1972.

Below: Early in the riot of July 17, 1972, ringleader Lascell "Cadillac" Gallop (below in white hat) stands with hostages Captain Clarence Davis, Charles Gilfuss, and Nathan Pashen (arms akimbo). Davis is handcuffed to Gilfuss, the handcuffs hidden from the camera by inmate Charles Creighton. The photograph was taken by Donald Shields, the ID officer, from wall post #1 at the end of the south wing. (Courtesy Capt. Robert L. Burrell.)

Right: The fire in the wood/metal shop (left) has been put out. Officials, one with a bullhorn, negotiate with inmates, who now hold the hostages on the fire escape of the Annapolis building. (Courtesy, Lt. James Felix.)

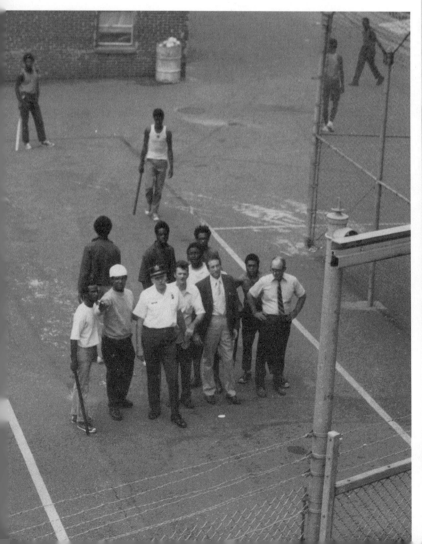

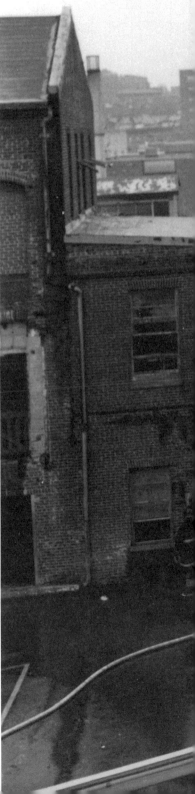

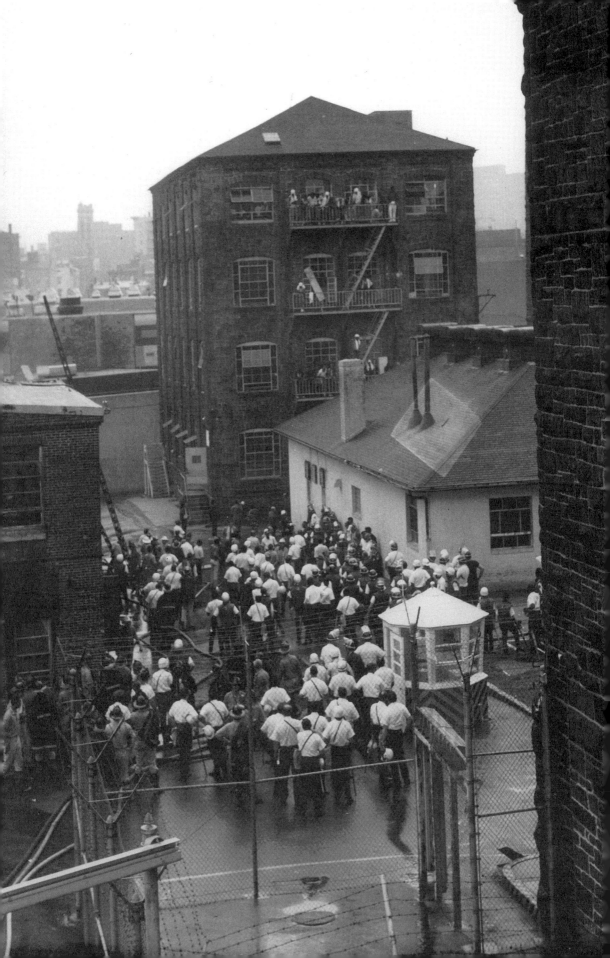

Prisoners vented their anger in the commissary, where the riot started (right and below), in the art/drawing room and library, both in the old Annapolis building (bottom left), and elsewhere. They also visited their wrath on an innocent barber's chair, and on a bell, symbol of what controlled their lives.

Overleaf: Firemen and riot control officers (in vests and helmets, with dogs) rest after putting out the fire in the wood/metal shop. (Photographs courtesy Lt. James Felix.)

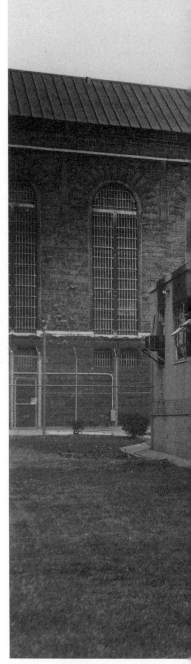

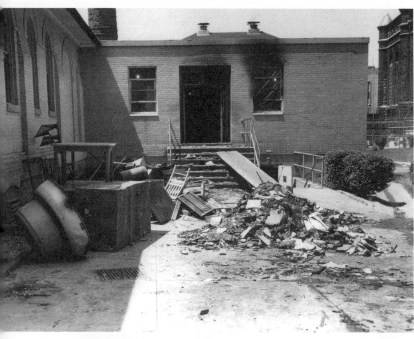

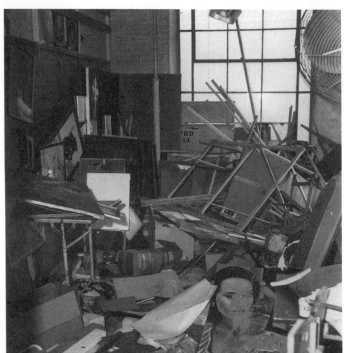

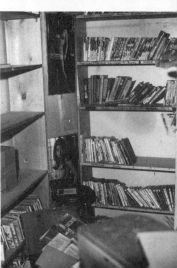

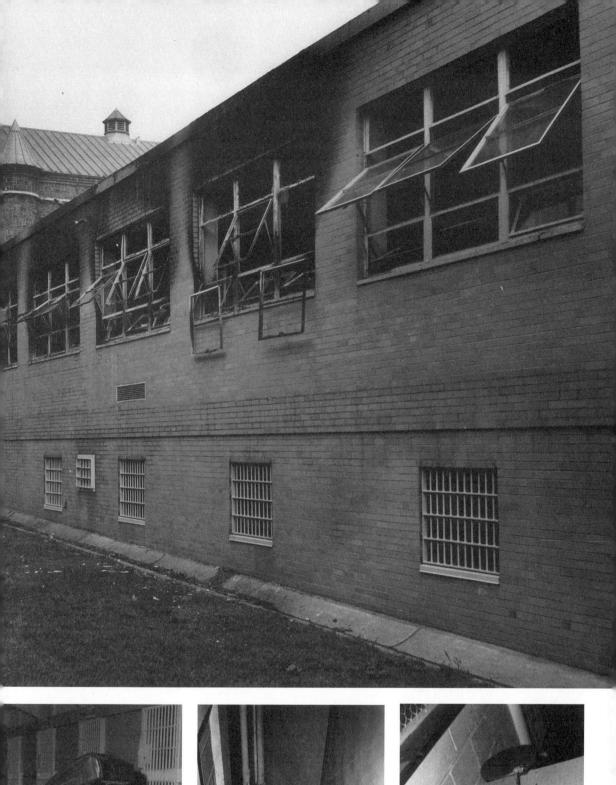
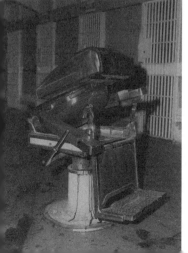
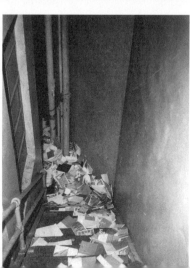
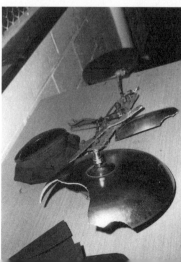

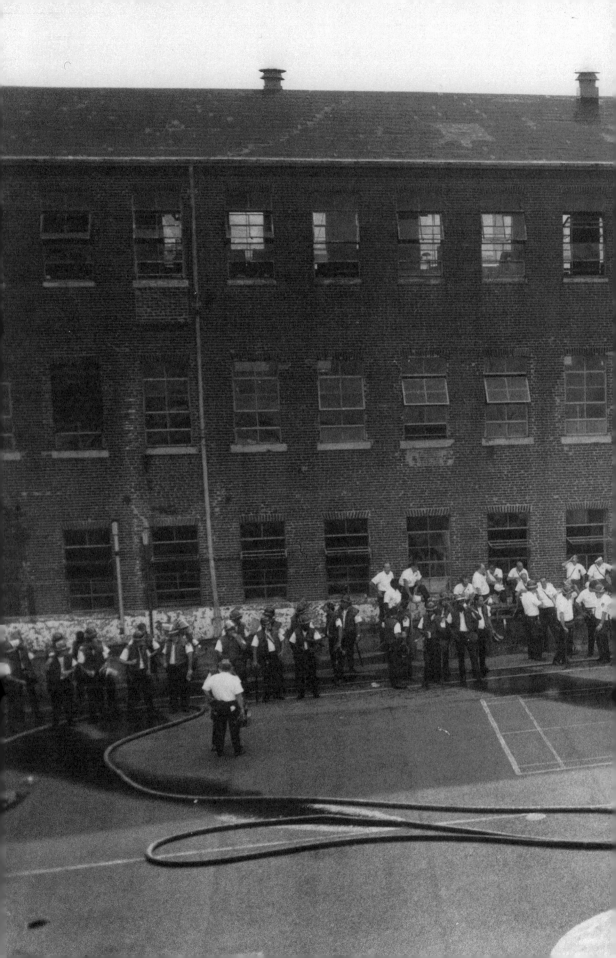

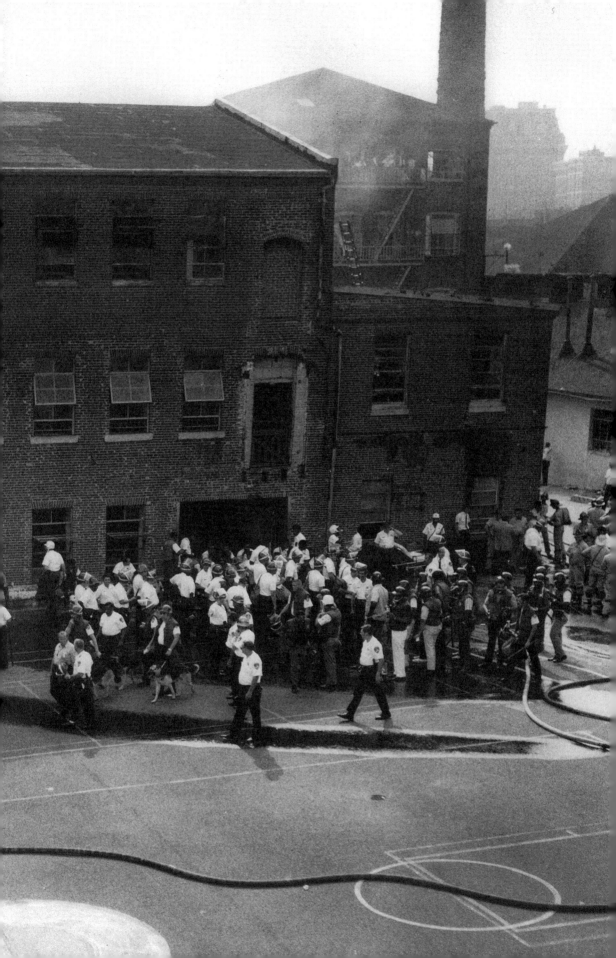

next serious riot. At 7:40 on a Friday evening, March 19, 1973, seventy-five prisoners took over the west wing in a spontaneous outbreak, erecting barricades and smashing out the lights. Seven guards were taken hostage; the rioters hanged two of them briefly before peaceful inmates saved them. Prisoners saved two more by dressing them in prison denims and pushing them into cells out the way of rampaging convicts. Correctional officers were able to restore order in only two hours because of the penitentiary's new riot control plan involving early response to prevent rioters from becoming well organized, a no-negotiations policy, and a policy of keeping out the news media. City police with K-9 dogs helped riot-trained guards use "divide and conquer" tactics on the dissident inmates. They used large quantities of incapacitating chemical spray, and fired two or three dozen non-lethal plastic bullets from ordinary shotguns. Three guards and three inmates were hospitalized and twenty-three inmates treated for cuts and bruises. Commissioner of Corrections James Jordan speculated that overcrowding might have contributed to the outbreak.[56]

Indeed, overcrowding in all Maryland prisons had increased alarmingly in recent months and would remain a serious problem for the rest of the decade and into the 1990s. Ever larger numbers of offenders were sent to prison by judges in response to the growing "get-tough" mood of the public.[57]

Meanwhile, despite the swift suppression of the March 19 riot, penitentiary inmates remained ready to take out their frustrations on correctional officers. At 6:20 P.M. on July 12, 1973, guard Jefferson O. Jackson was attacked by five inmates in the south wing in retribution for having placed an inmate in solitary for a rules violation. Jackson was stabbed in the neck, throat, and chest and hospitalized in critical condition. A second officer, Barron E. Burch, suffered cuts and bruises. City police were ordered to the prison in case a riot developed, but a group of guards forcibly put down the disturbance. Two weeks later, the five rebellious inmates filed suit in federal court for $17.5 million, saying guards had beaten them and violated their civil rights. Representatives from the Black Panther Party and the George Jackson Prison Movement raised money and drummed up community support for "the Maryland Pen 5," but four years later a federal jury ruled in favor of prison officials.[58]

The day after the stabbing of Officer Jackson, a hundred guards met with Warden Gerald H. McClellan and demanded that the metal shop be closed

---

[56]"75 Run Rampant," *Baltimore News-American,* March 30, 1973, "Guards Free Seven Hostages, End 2-Hour Riot At Md. Pen," and "New Riot Plan Used At Pen," *Baltimore Evening Sun,* March 30, 1973.

[57]"Prison Population in Maryland rises to 'intolerable' level," *Baltimore News-American,* January 3, 1973.

[58]"Two Guards Injured in Prison Attack," *Baltimore News-American,* July 13, 1973; "5 Inmates Ask $17.5 Million in Pen Suit," *Baltimore News-American,* July 27, 1973; and "5 at Pen Alleging Official Brutality Lose Damage Suit," *Baltimore Sun,* September 22, 1977.

down, to reduce inmates' ability to make weapons, such as knives. Some threat-ened to go on strike until the warden met their demand. McClellan complied. If prisoners at this time were becoming more conscious of their so-called rights and ready to fight for them, so were the guards. It was not a pleasant situation for any warden to be in, though it had nothing to do with McClellan's resigna-tion, for "personal reasons," less than a year later. His successor, veteran captain George H. Collins, became the penitentiary's first black warden on October 9, 1974.[59] He would hold the post throughout nine difficult years, the sixth long-est tenure of any warden in the penitentiary's history.

Collins inherited the serious problem of overcrowding, which for nearly two years had been especially acute in the penitentiary's west wing and resulted in double-celling there in over half the cells. Only twenty-six shower heads were available for 837 men—"we run the showers day and night," said one guard captain. Prisoners had only ten to fifteen minutes in which to eat their meals, crammed together twenty to a table in the old dining hall. The penitentiary also lacked a gymnasium and other recreational facilities, and the resulting bore-dom and frustration had turned the institution into a pressure cooker.[60]

To relieve overcrowding throughout the correctional system, Commissioner James Jordan called for construction of more prisons, but the governor and leg-islature were reluctant to commit the funds. Community correctional centers, similar to "half-way" houses, were also sought to reduce the prison population, but people living in the designated neighborhoods opposed them. For a time in 1976, the state seriously considered converting a mothballed Navy troop ship into a floating minimum-security prison anchored in the Canton area of Baltimore's harbor, but the idea died in the face of neighborhood opposition.[61]

Time was running out. On January 25, 1977, the Baltimore Legal Aid Bu-reau filed the first of several suits on behalf of penitentiary inmates to end over-crowding. The penitentiary now held 1,500 prisoners, it charged, twice the intended capacity, and consequently conditions were deplorable. The facility lacked sanitation and space for recreational, educational, or training programs and had developed an atmosphere of violence and brutality. A representative of the Legal Aid Bureau called for increased use of parole and probation and com-munity corrections centers to reduce the prison population.[62]

---

[59]"State Penitentiary Metal Shop Is Closed in Bid to Cut Weapon-Making by Inmates," *Baltimore Sun,* July 14, 1973; "McClellan Quits as Warden," *Baltimore News-American,* March 29, 1974. Confirmed by inter-view with retired warden Gerald H. McClellan, April 28, 1995. "Two Top Prison Positions Are Filled by Appointment from State Roster," *Baltimore Sun,* October 9, 1974.

[60]"Prison Population in Maryland Rises to 'intolerable' level," *Baltimore News-American,* January 3, 1973.

[61]"New State Prisons Urged," *Baltimore News-American,* January 4, 1973; "'Mothballed' Troop Ship to be a Maryland Prison," *Baltimore News-American,* May 20, 1976; and "Prison Ship Opposed in Canton Area," *Baltimore News-American,* October 15, 1976.

[62]"Conditions Assailed as Suit Urges Pen's Closing," *Baltimore Sun,* January 26, 1977.

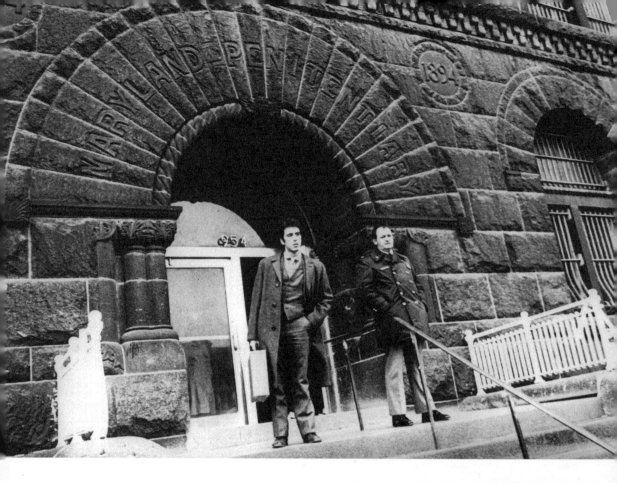

Above: A publicity still for the film *And Justice for All* (1979). Actor Al Pacino stands at the penitentiary entrance with Major Svend Hansen.

Right: Comedian Redd Foxx entertained inmates in the early 1970s. (Photographs courtesy Lt. James Felix.)

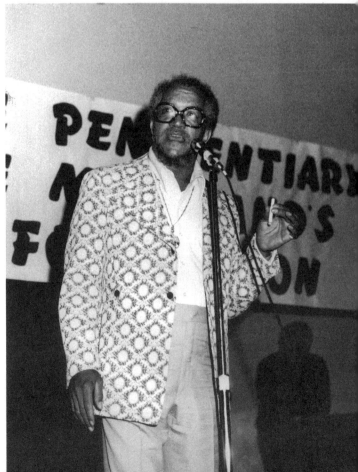

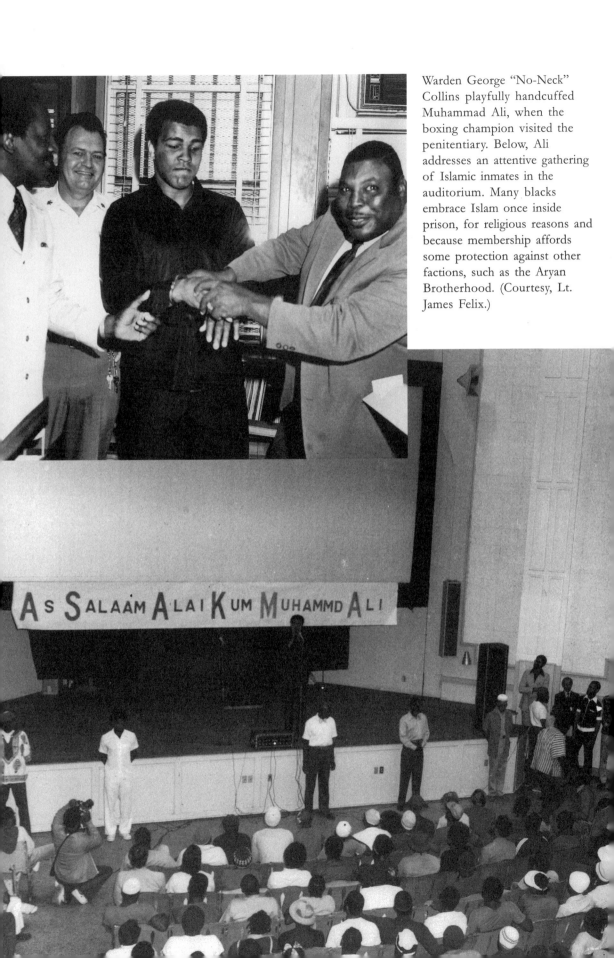

Warden George "No-Neck" Collins playfully handcuffed Muhammad Ali, when the boxing champion visited the penitentiary. Below, Ali addresses an attentive gathering of Islamic inmates in the auditorium. Many blacks embrace Islam once inside prison, for religious reasons and because membership affords some protection against other factions, such as the Aryan Brotherhood. (Courtesy, Lt. James Felix.)

As Salaam Alaikum Muhammd Ali

Community corrections centers—newly fashionable in official penology across the nation during the 1970s[63]—had been in the planning stage in Maryland since the fall of 1972. Their aim was to integrate the offender into the community as he approached the completion of his sentence. Small residential centers housing between seventy-five and a hundred persons each would be established throughout Baltimore City and the state in locations close to the area from which the offenders came. The facilities would be designed for normal residency living, with doors instead of bars and small tables for informal dining. For approximately four months the resident would participate during the day in vocational or educational training under close supervision. If his resulting adjustment record was positive, he would then be allowed to live at home for two months prior to his parole or release. The state had scheduled twelve of these centers to be built by 1983.[64]

But swifter action was needed. The suit to end overcrowding resulted in a federal court decree on January 24, 1979, ordering officials to reduce the penitentiary's population to 1,028 by October 1, 1980.[65]

In January 1979 newly elected Governor Harry R. Hughes chose a controversial figure from within the prison system, Gordon C. Kamka, to serve as Secretary of Public Safety and Correction Services with the hope that he could solve the overcrowding crisis. The relatively young Kamka (he was but thirty-nine years old), warden of the City Jail and a psychologist by training, believed strongly in establishing community correctional centers and the increased use of probation and parole to reduce the prison population. His nomination was opposed from the outset by such conservatives as Anne Arundel County Executive Robert Pascal and Chief Judge Robert C. Murphy of the state's Court of Appeals.[66] Pascal, especially, became a "self-styled Paul Revere" warning legislators and the citizenry about Kamka's lenient policies. In particular, he criticized Kamka's early-release program, which, he charged, freed armed robbers, rapists, and murderers, thereby endangering the lives of citizens.[67] The well-publicized arrest of Wendell Beard for murder while serving in a work-release

---

[63]Sullivan, *The Prison Reform Movement,* pp. 112–13.

[64]William E. Lamb, Community Corrections Task Force, "Correction Centers Offer Jobs," *Maryland Division of Correction Newsletter* (September 1972): 5, and "Cannon Assails State Role," *Baltimore Sun,* September 29, 1972.

[65]"State Just Meets Deadline on Prison Overcrowding," *Baltimore Sun,* October 1, 1980.

[66]"The Man Hughes Wants to Run the Maryland Prison System," and "Kamka: Fewer Prisoners, Not More Prisons," *Baltimore News-American,* (clipping in Division of Correction files, not dated, but published shortly after Kamka's appointment on January 17, 1979); "Hughes Takes Risk with New Approach to Prison Problem," *Baltimore Sun,* February 25, 1979.

[67]"Pascal's Opposition to Prison Policies of Hughes Called an Obsession," *Baltimore Sun,* September 3,

program helped substantiate Pascal's charges. By the spring of 1981, criticism of Kamka's prison policies had grown to the point that both he and his hand-picked commissioner of corrections, Edwin R. Goodlander, were forced to re-sign on March 30.[68]

This turmoil in the Maryland prison system, caused by conflicting conservative and liberal prison philosophies, was called "a dramatic example of a national debate between those who believe in punishment and building more jails and those who favor alternatives to incarceration because they believe that imprisonment alone will not affect crime." Governor Hughes had learned a lesson from his failed experiment in liberal penology. In Maryland, the mood of the public was swinging now toward reaction and repression, along with the rest of the nation.[69] The resulting "lock 'em up" mentality would inevitably worsen overcrowding at the penitentiary.

1979, and "New Hughes: Firm on Prison Policy," *Baltimore News-American* (clipping in Division of Correction files undated, but content suggests publication in fall 1979).

[68]"3 Charged in City Murder," *Baltimore Sun,* September 5, 1979; "Kamka, Before He Quit, Resumed Work-Release," *Baltimore News-American,* April 2, 1981.

[69]"In Maryland, a Conflict Over Prison Philosophies," *New York Times,* September 25, 1982; Sullivan, *The Prison Reform Movement,* chapter seven, "Reaction and Repression: The 1980s."

Overleaf: Aerial view of the penitentiary, ca. 1979, looking south. (Courtesy, Lt. James Felix.)

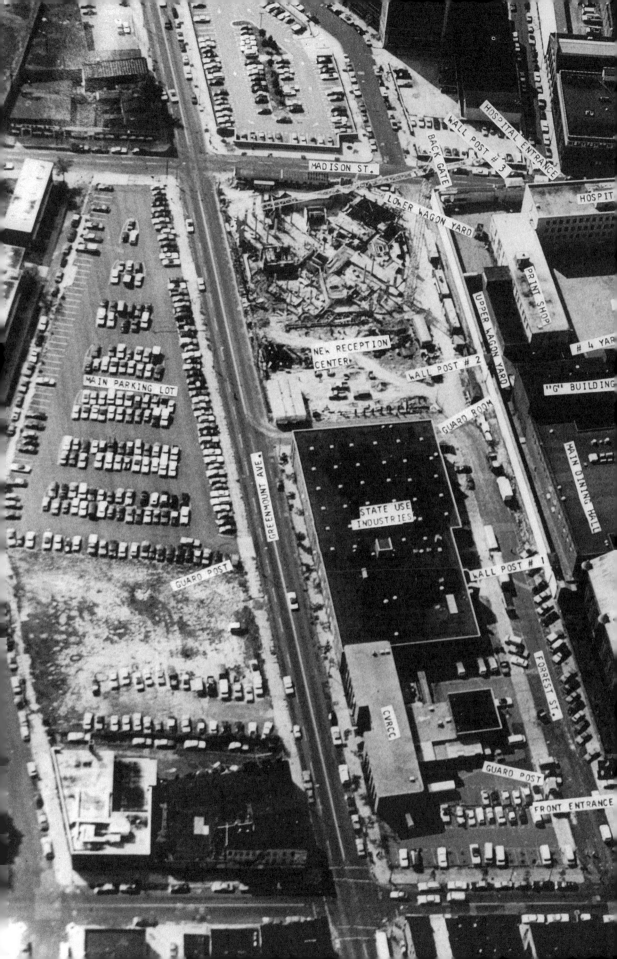

MADISON ST.

HOSPITAL ENTRANCE

WALL POST # 3

BACK GATE

HOSPIT

LOWER WAGON YARD

PRINT SHOP

4 YAR

NEW RECEPTION CENTER

UPPER WAGON YARD

WALL POST # 2

"G" BUILDING

MAIN PARKING LOT

GUARD ROOM

MAIN DINING HALL

GREENMOUNT AVE.

STATE USE INDUSTRIES

WALL POST # 1

GUARD POST

FORREST ST.

CVRCC

GUARD POST

FRONT ENTRANCE

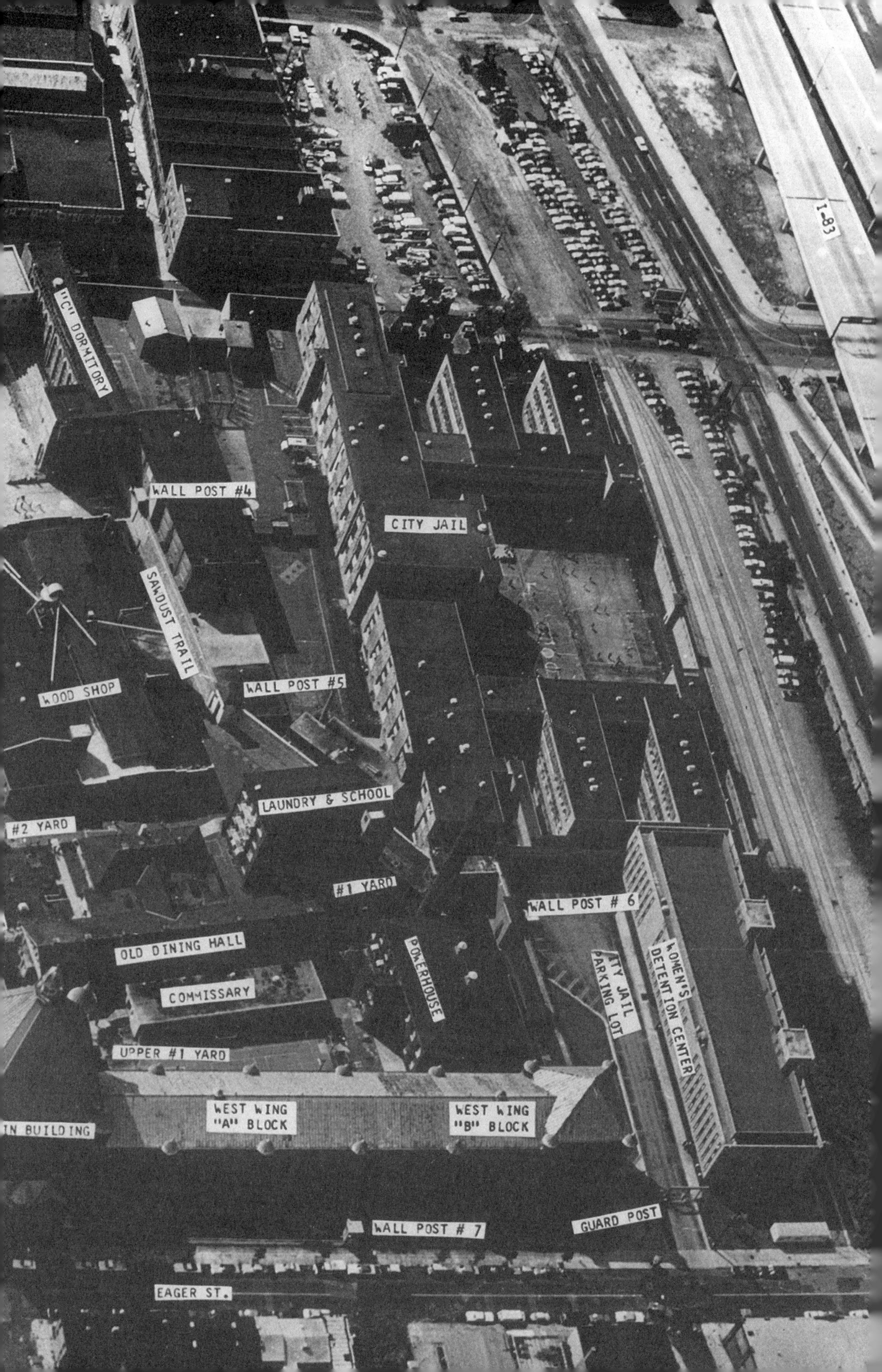

"C" DORMITORY

WALL POST #4

CITY JAIL

I-83

SAWDUST TRAIL

WOOD SHOP

WALL POST #5

#2 YARD

LAUNDRY & SCHOOL

#1 YARD

WALL POST # 6

OLD DINING HALL

POWERHOUSE

COMMISSARY

CITY JAIL PARKING LOT

WOMEN'S DETENTION CENTER

UPPER #1 YARD

IN BUILDING

WEST WING "A" BLOCK

WEST WING "B" BLOCK

WALL POST # 7

GUARD POST

EAGER ST.

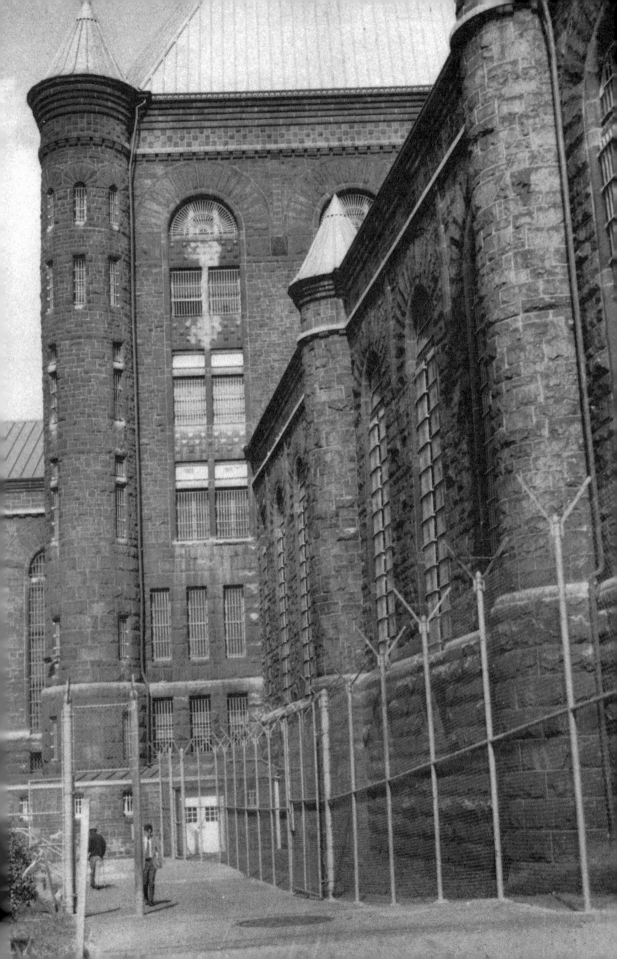

Chapter Seven

Keeping the Lid On

1981 – 1995

"Politicians ultimately control the system, and they will always reflect the public's attitude toward crime. And that attitude now says to lock up criminals."
—Larry E. Sullivan, *The Prison Reform Movement: Forlorn Hope* (1990)

Overcrowding at the Maryland Penitentiary, as elsewhere, raised tensions among inmates and between them and the guards, turning it into a potentially explosive cauldron. Without adequate staff to supervise inmates, prison officials were forced to reduce recreation and rehabilitation programs. Prisoners became bored and restless and resentful, increasingly ready to assault each other or the guards and to riot or try to escape. Early in 1981, the dangerous working conditions even caused twenty-five guards to call in sick rather than report for duty,[1] which of course only worsened the problem. Overcrowding would continue to plague the entire prison system throughout the 1980s and into the 1990s, and penitentiary administrators, along with others, would struggle, not always with success, to keep the lid on, until the final act was played out in the penitentiary's historic role as the state's only maximum-security prison.

In choosing a new Secretary of Public Safety and Correctional Services, Governor Harry Hughes sought to improve his reëlection prospects by appointing hard-liner Thomas W. Schmidt, a veteran state bureaucrat, in April 1981. Schmidt won the approval of conservative legislators and did much to calm the public's outrage over his predecessor's liberal penal philosophy by tightening up the pre-release program and stopping early paroles. He quickly resumed double-celling (putting two inmates in a cell designed for one) to compensate

---

[1]"Penitentiary guards call in sick to protest 'dangerous working conditions,'" *Baltimore Sun,* February 28, 1981.

Opposite: The prison administration building and south wing (on right) in the 1980s. The photograph was taken from inside the #1 yard. (Courtesy, Capt. Robert Lee Burrell.)

195

for the resulting backup in the prison pipeline. Fortunately for the new secretary, two prisons would open in 1981—a 512-bed facility at Jessup and the 400-bed Reception-Diagnostic & Classification Center near the penitentiary—and offer some relief from the problem of overcrowding, not only at the penitentiary but throughout the prison system. But in response to the public's call for safer streets, judges were handing out more prison sentences, and the problem of overcrowding would soon return.[2]

The resumption of double-celling in the Maryland prison system, despite a federal court order prohibiting it, was therefore an unsatisfactory expedient. More prisons would be needed, but for political reasons legislators were unwilling to vote for the necessary funds or to offend their constituents by building those prisons in their own cities and counties.[3]

Meanwhile, two successful escapes from the penitentiary in eleven days resulted in embarrassing publicity for prison officials. The first escape occurred on April 11, 1982, Easter Sunday, when two inmates on janitorial duty in the penitentiary's lobby overpowered two guards in the control booth, opened the front door, and walked out with a third inmate. Then on April 22, two inmates overpowered the maintenance supervisor of a work detail in the prison hospital, took over a welding torch, and burned through the bars to freedom. In both escapes, prison officials blamed correctional officers, but a union representative defended them, saying, "There's more people in the prisons and too few people to watch them."[4]

Dangerous working conditions at the overcrowded penitentiary were again publicized on September 25, 1982, when seventeen guards at the neighboring Reception-Diagnostic & Classification Center refused their assignment inside the penitentiary's crowded F-block (an old converted wood shop), saying they felt ill and unable to work.[5] Negotiations at the penitentiary between corrections chief Schmidt, who wanted to dismiss the guards, and union officials were interrupted by an escape attempt on September 28, during which three inmates scaled the penitentiary's west wall and took two guards hostage before being put down in a bloody shoot-out with other guards.[6] By now it was clear to the public that new, up-to-date facilities and work-rehabilitation programs were needed for Maryland's exploding prison population.[7]

---

[2]"Quiet bureaucrat brings tough regime to prisons," *Baltimore Sun,* September 7, 1981.

[3]"Maryland's double-celling controversy: 'We're losing control,'" *Baltimore News-American,* May 7, 1981.

[4]"Pen escapers are recaptured within minutes," and "Galley sets Pen study after rash of escapes," *Baltimore Sun,* April 23, 1982.

[5]"Reception guards facing Pen duty return to work," *Baltimore Evening Sun,* September 24, 1982, and "Dispute over prison staffing appears to continue," *Baltimore Sun,* September 25, 1982.

[6]"5 wounded in shoot-out at state Pen," *Baltimore Sun,* September 29, 1982, and "Trouble at the state penitentiary," *Baltimore News-American,* September 29, 1982.

[7]"Maryland's Prison Problem," *Baltimore Sun,* editorial, September 29, 1982.

By the spring of 1983, funding for new prison construction had been approved, and federal judge Alexander Harvey II ruled that overcrowding at the penitentiary could continue until the new permanent facilities were completed. In rendering his decision, Harvey said the failure of prison officials to solve the overcrowding problem was due to "unprecedented increases in the number of prisoners coming into the Maryland system during the past two years."[8] Indeed, a U.S. Department of Justice bulletin revealed a record increase in the nation's prison population in those years—a 11.6 percent increase in 1982 and a 12.2 percent increase the year before—together, the largest growth since 1925, when records were first kept. Part of this growth the bulletin attributed to post–World War II male baby boomers, who were reaching crime-prone years. But it also cited tough new sentencing laws and tighter parole policies across the country in response to growing public pressure to keep criminals in prison longer.[9]

For the Maryland prison system, the 1983 statistics proved alarming. The average length of stay in prison had almost doubled since the mid-1970s to about two years. Maryland's prison population had reached almost thirteen thousand—already exceeding in 1983 the predicted figure for 1990—and was growing at the rate of 125 inmates a month. Although new construction would add 2,200 more beds by 1987, Maryland prisons were expected to be 30 percent over capacity at that time. Prison costs were calculated by experts as follows: $70,000 per cell to construct a prison, $15,000 to keep an inmate a year, plus hidden costs of lost taxes, welfare for his family, his unpaid bills. Fringe benefits for prison staff could double the annual maintenance cost. Construction costs could more than triple if interest paid on the debt was included.[10] Small wonder that construction of new, modern prisons could not keep up with the need for them. The lid was about to blow.

Violence erupted on October 6, 1984, in the penitentiary's notorious south wing, a segregation unit for the most unruly inmates. At 3 P.M., three inmates being led back to their cells after an exercise period stabbed four guards, killing one and wounding three. The dead officer, Herman Toulson Jr., was the first guard killed on duty in nearly sixty years.[11] But other, non-fatal attacks on south wing staff had occurred earlier, and all of the penitentiary guards were well

---

[8]"Judge OKs crowding at Penitentiary," *Baltimore Sun*, March 3, 1983. Judge Harvey was being more lenient here than two years earlier: "Judge to 'personally monitor' prison cell limits," *Baltimore Evening Sun*, January 6, 1981.

[9]"Record increase in federal, state prison population," *Baltimore Afro-American*, April 30, 1983.

[10]"Crowding escalates in prisons—Tensions threaten life in Penitentiary, symposium hears," *Baltimore Sun*, February 27, 1984.

[11]"Guard killed, several hurt in Pen fracas," *Baltimore Sun*, October 7, 1984. The first guard ever to be killed in the line of duty was Robert H. Holtman, who was struck with an iron pipe by escapee Richard Whittemore on February 20, 1925, and died two days later. I owe this observation to a recent unpublished historical sketch, "A Penitentiary for the Free State" (1995), by inmate Paul Inskeep (#211-806), p. 19.

aware of its dangerous working conditions. Toulson himself, after six years' duty there, had requested a transfer in June, complaining of verbal threats as well as urine and feces being thrown on him by some of the inmates. Both that request and another were denied.

Toulson's death and the injuries to the other guards resulted in meetings held by the correctional officers' unions. They called for the resignation of Warden Leslie H. Dorsey, charging him with understaffing the south wing and failing to heed their warnings of trouble there.[12] Although forbidden by law to strike, they began a sick-out job action that ended only when state officials promised to probe security conditions in the south wing.[13]

Some individual correctional officers spoke out, too, blaming violence at the penitentiary on the recent reforms in treatment of inmates. According to one veteran guard, who chose to remain anonymous, prisoners were more willing to attack guards since the penitentiary's unofficial "goon squad"—a group of physically large guards who dispensed retaliatory beatings—had been done away with by prison administrators a decade earlier.[14] Retired lieutenant Richard Powers reached back further, blaming the "new idea" (liberal) policies introduced by Joseph G. Cannon, appointed Commissioner of Corrections in 1967. The new system, Powers said, had upset the mutual survival accommodation between prisoners and the old style, experienced line guards, a sense of "how far men and events could go—or would be permitted to go." The new style administrators, he continued, had lost touch with life on the tiers: "I'll bet my last dollar that a review of the south wing activities over the 30 days preceding Officer Toulson's death will find evidence reeking with danger signals. Signs the administration was unable to read or unable to counter."[15]

His prediction was amply borne out. Two months later, a 142-page report compiled by Attorney General Stephen H. Sachs made newspaper headlines. Calling the penitentiary's south wing "the innermost circle of Hell in the Maryland prison system," it described in vivid detail the living and security conditions there. "The South Wing is noisy and filthy. A constant racket reverberates and echoes in the granite building. It smells of urine, vomit, rotting food and body odor. . . . There are pigeon droppings on nearly every flat surface. . . . Assaults and stabbings are an everyday occurrence. Contraband—drugs and weapons—flows in a stream of illicit commerce from cell to cell and tier to tier.

---

[12]"Guard slain in prison sought transfer in June," *Baltimore Sun,* October 8, 1984, and "Union asks pen warden to resign," *Baltimore Evening Sun,* October 8, 1984.

[13]"Pen guards end sick-out after probe pledge," *Baltimore Evening Sun,* October 15, 1984.

[14]"Guard Slain in Prison Sought Transfer in June," *Baltimore Sun,* October 8, 1984.

[15]Richard Powers, "The delicate balance of prison life," *Baltimore Evening Sun,* October 17, 1984.

Inmate-set fires are daily events. . . . For the first nine months of this year, there were 26 serious-incident reports involving inmate-upon-inmate violence . . . 13 serious-incident reports of inmate assaults on officers." The physical plant and layout were obsolete, the equipment (doors and locks, phones, two-way radios) undependable. Although the Sachs report said these conditions resulted from years of administrative mismanagement and neglect, it also blamed Warden Dorsey, his assistant warden, and the chief of security for being "virtual strangers to the day-to-day operations of the South Wing." Governor Hughes ordered the immediate transfer of the warden and his aides and the implementation of most of the report's thirty recommendations for security and staffing improvements. The Sachs report would prove a catalyst for some much-needed changes.[16]

Most conspicuous was the proposal to construct a three-hundred-bed, super maximum-security prison to replace the penitentiary's decrepit south wing segregation unit. Demolition work began to clear a lot across Madison Street opposite the penitentiary for the new "Supermax."[17] The site had been chosen after some debate and not without neighborhood residents objecting to yet another prison being put in their backyard.[18]

But one year after Officer Toulson's death, the penitentiary's south wing, despite some improvement, continued to experience problems.[19] More inmate assaults on guards occurred.[20] And over the years, the steel cellblocks standing within its granite walls had become badly rusted from numerous floodings by inmates who stopped up their toilets and then flushed them repeatedly. Now the whole structure threatened to collapse. Sensing this, the inmates—after an audio-signal—would create additional stress by jumping up and down in cadence.[21] The completion of the Supermax would come none too soon.

To the dismay of corrections officials, the flow of inmates into the Maryland system continued to outpace the construction of new prisons, as judges—

---

[16]"Pen's warden ousted after prison report," *Baltimore Sun,* November 14, 1984; "Hughes orders slash in Pen double-celling," *Baltimore Evening Sun,* November 14, 1984; and "Prisons chief promises to fix up Pen," *Baltimore Sun,* November 15, 1984.

[17]"Will 'supermax' be free of drugs?" *Baltimore Evening Sun,* November 8, 1985.

[18]"High-rise prison for 300 near Pen sought by Hughes," *Baltimore Sun,* January 22, 1985; "Hopkins defends city site for new 'super' prison," *Baltimore Evening Sun,* February 12, 1985; and "Mitchell leads protest against putting prison at East Baltimore site," *Baltimore Sun,* February 24, 1985.

[19]"Problems persist in cleaned-up prison," *Baltimore Evening Sun,* October 4, 1985; "Pen makes changes, but major flaws remain," *Baltimore Sun,* October 6, 1985; and "Improved South Wing remains a Hell," *Baltimore Sun,* April 11, 1986.

[20]"Guard stabbed by convict at Penitentiary," *Baltimore Sun,* April 3, 1986, and "Pen guard stabbed by inmates," *Baltimore Sun,* April 19, 1986.

[21]"Officials Fear Pen Wing Could Collapse," *Baltimore Sun,* November 3, 1988. The penitentiary's audit coordinator, Andrew Stritch, recalls: "The signal would be one inmate yelling, 'Was your food cold today?' 'Yeah!' came the answer. Then they would all begin jumping up and down together with a heavy metallic bass sound, like ten cars hitting all at once." (Interview, October 14, 1992).

responding to the public's call to "get tough"—committed more and more offenders, mainly for drug-related crimes as a cocaine and "crack" epidemic took hold. Without adequate job training and basic education to sustain them, 40 percent of all inmates returned to prison within three years. In November 1987, newly appointed public safety secretary Bishop L. Robinson brought forth a comprehensive eleven-year plan to stop this revolving door phenomenon and thereby reduce overcrowding. Among other things, Robinson called for a new building program that stressed the rehabilitation of prisoners. Its main proposal called for the construction of two pre-release centers—one in Baltimore, the other in Prince George's County—to provide job skills and basic education and to treat the nearly 70 percent of inmates with drug problems. Robinson's plan was ambitious and expensive. It would take some time to get the backing of Governor William Donald Schaefer's administration and the public.[22]

In the interim, bad news lay ahead for any guards who might still believe in a "goon squad" to even the score with violent inmates. On January 29, 1988, over four years after the south wing fracas that resulted in the death of officer Herman Toulson Jr., eight penitentiary guards were indicted in federal court over the retaliatory beatings of Toulson's killer, Nathaniel Appleby, and two other inmates. Ultimately, six of them would be convicted for violating the civil rights of the three inmates.[23] This highly visible case would serve as a warning to correctional officers throughout Maryland's prison system who might be tempted in the future to take justice into their own hands.

More embarrassing headlines followed. Inside the overcrowded penitentiary, the usual random violence—one inmate stabbing or beating up another—was broken on July 25, 1988, by the first riot in fifteen years, which started with three separate and nearly simultaneous attacks on guards. If prison officials did not know something would happen that Monday, most of the inmates clearly did. Only forty-five of the usual three hundred came to the dining hall for the noon "feed-up." The rest stayed in their cells on a food strike, either because they did not wish to become involved or because they had been told to stay out of trouble by those who had planned the riot.[24]

The first fight began in yard #4 at the southern end of the penitentiary complex. At 12:45 P.M., Corporal Robert Baysmore entered the guard shack to answer the phone and was attacked from behind by Kenneth Mack-Bey (#178-

---

[22]"Opening Up the Doors to Prison Reform," *Baltimore Sun,* November 1, 1987, and "Landmark Prison Plan," *Baltimore Sun,* November 8, 1987.

[23]"U.S. indicts 8 Pen guards in beatings," *Baltimore Sun,* January 29, 1988, and "6 Pen guards convicted in rights case tied to beating," *Baltimore Evening Sun,* July 8, 1988.

[24]The account of this riot is based on penitentiary files and a newspaper account, "9 of Pen staff hurt in riot," *Baltimore Sun,* July 26, 1988.

594) and stabbed over the left eye. While Baysmore grappled with Mack-Bey, he was attacked by Kenneth Pasco (#177-313), Jeffrey ("World") Coates (#176-291), Derek Davis (#180-932), and George Willoughby (#167-793) wielding pipes and baseball bats. Lieutenant James V. Peguese ran to help Baysmore but was beaten to the ground, suffering a broken nose and shoulder blade, and multiple bruises.

The second fight occurred minutes later in yard #3. Glen Jones (#171-544), Robert Smallwood (#163-669), Ronald Cunningham (#173-396), Dennis Wise (#153-205), and other inmates wielding pipes, baseball bats, and knives attacked Corporal Russell Biddle and Corporal James Hawkins. Elsewhere, Officer Kevin Atkins had both his arms broken and was beaten all over his body with bats by Donald Griffin (#175-236), Michael ("Food Stamps") Stewart (#175-252), Donald Braxton (#163-023), and Michael ("Little Black Ass") Mouzone (#152-182). Meanwhile, penitentiary officials and a tactical force armed with riot batons, mace, and shotguns responded to radio calls for help from officers on the hospital roof and wall. A warning shot into the air, ordered by Major Theodore Purnell, accidentally wounded officer Antoine Givens in the neck on #4 wall post.

The last fight came when inmates rushed the crisis clinic in the hospital building at the south end of yard #4, trashing and setting fire to an office. They assaulted Corporal Evetral Fielder, lacerating her head and neck, and psychologist Joseph Fuhrmaneck, who suffered a broken ankle and multiple head and facial wounds. At 1:20 P.M. a team of officers headed by Assistant Warden Sewall Smith entered the clinic through the rear and met inmates Wyman Ushery (#173-796) and Anthony Hughley (#190-065) advancing with a knife and a piece of metal. Ordered to drop their weapons, they refused and were stopped by a single shotgun blast that wounded both. Smith then continued into the yard where hundreds of inmates were milling about and brought them under control. So ended a riot that sent eight correctional officers, three inmates, and a prison psychologist to local hospitals but resulted in no escapes and no hostages taken.

In the aftermath, disciplinary charges were brought against thirty-eight inmates and criminal charges against nine. Exactly who might have planned the riot and why is unclear. Anonymous letters from inmates to officials in the prison files mention, variously, discontent among Muslim inmates, a grievance by the Inmate Advisory Council over new clothing and property regulations, the urging of the Monday food strike at a prison NAACP meeting the previous Saturday, and a plan by a group of older inmates to "buck up" (incite) the "hoppers" (younger inmates) into attacking the guards in yards #3 and #4 and escape in the ensuing confusion. Representatives of the correctional officers' union blamed the prison administration for ignoring the clear warning of trouble, signaled by the food strike.

Some relief for correctional officers working in the dangerous conditions of the penitentiary's south wing was expected with the opening of the new segregation facility, the Maryland Correctional Adjustment Center, in January 1989. Built at a cost of $21 million, the 288-cell super-maximum-security facility, more popularly known as Supermax, would serve as a prison for the most violent inmates within the prison system. In designing its exterior, the architectural firm of George W. Bushey in Hagerstown departed from the two-hundred-year-old tradition of the prison fortress look, intended to awe or intimidate the passerby. Unlike the old granite penitentiary, Supermax has clean modern lines and is built of light brown brick. No guard towers are visible, no tinsel rolls of razor ribbon are to be seen over its walls. Across the main entrance plaza, the stylish dark glass façade of its administration building suggests that of a prosperous suburban bank.[25]

A circular design for the cell houses was chosen to allow maximum supervision of inmates with a minimum of custodial manpower. Whereas the old penitentiary's rectangular, steel cage cellblocks required numerous correctional officers to supervise the straight rows of cells, Supermax has centrally located control booths surrounded by cells. The 288 individual cells are divided equally among a row of three octagonal two-story cell houses and located in their peripheries, thus falling under the surveillance of central control booths.

The details of cell construction were carefully thought out for maximum security. The cell walls are poured concrete, eight inches thick and reinforced with steel rods. Much of the seven-by-ten-foot floor space is taken up by a concrete-slab bed to the left, topped with a light-green vinyl mattress containing flame-resistant material. To the right of the cell door in a slanted corner (to prevent an inmate from surprising a guard) is a stainless steel toilet-sink combination operated by pushbuttons. The toilet has a "floodbuster" valve set for only three consecutive flushes, to discourage the inmate from flooding the cell. The light fixture over the sink has a shock-and-chip resistant lens and a built-in intercom, which can monitor cell noise. The mirror set in the wall is stainless steel. In the far corner is a small shelf desk of quarter-inch steel and a stool bolted to the floor. Three clothes hooks bolted to the wall are each on a pivot and spring loaded to prevent the inmate from hanging himself. The cell windows

---

[25]Details about Supermax came from a tour of the facility and interview with its architects, the George W. Bushey firm in Hagerstown, Maryland, in December 1988.

are narrow (six inches high and fourteen inches wide) to prevent the inmate from squeezing through.[26]

Even with the opening of two new prisons within two years—the Eastern Correctional Institution in Somerset County and Supermax—the State of Maryland could not keep up with the flow of inmates into the prison system. In the ten months ending April 30, 1989, the total prison population jumped by more than 950 to 14,268, which was 22 percent over the system's functioning capacity of 11,681 inmates. The acute need for more prison beds threatened the state's plan to scrap and replace the obsolete Maryland Penitentiary and House of Correction and forced prison officials to think about opening up areas of prison buildings not originally intended to house inmates. But even as they considered this emergency measure, prison officials were being held accountable by such inmate advocacy groups as the American Civil Liberties Union National Prison Project and Legal Aid Bureau Prison Assistance Project, who wanted the number and type of prisoners housed there restricted.[27] Such political pressures made it increasingly difficult for prison officials—including those at the penitentiary— to keep the population of each facility under court-approved numerical ceilings.

Two long-term solutions to overcrowding seemed to offer some hope. The first was placing non-violent offenders under house arrest (with the help of electronic monitoring technology) or using similar alternatives to imprisonment. The other, favored by Maryland's public safety secretary Bishop L. Robinson, emphasized rehabilitation programs—in the belief that given job and social skills before reentry into society, prisoners would be less likely to repeat their crimes—and closer supervision of parolees, including financial aid if they fell ill or lost their job and were in danger of lapsing into crime. A key part of Robinson's plan to prepare prisoners for reentry into society would be the construction of a new Metropolitan Transition Services Center at the Maryland Penitentiary to supervise those soon to be released.[28]

While public safety secretary Robinson tried to deal with the prison system's overcrowding problem, the penitentiary experienced another riot. Unlike the riot of July 25, 1988, penitentiary officials received a tip on July 15, 1991, that a diversionary disturbance would be followed by an escape attempt planned for that week. They took what precautions they could. Tactical units in the area

---

[26]And yet, that is exactly what slender (5 feet 11 inches, 145 lbs.) Harold Benjamin Dean managed to do on November 30, 1991, the first escape from Supermax ("Killer makes first escape from 'Supermax,'" *Baltimore Sunday Sun*, December 1, 1991). He was recaptured ten months later ("FBI finds killer in Ohio town," *Baltimore Sun*, October 2, 1992).

[27]"Prison growth outpaced by new inmates," *Baltimore Sun*, April 30, 1989.

[28]"Prison Puzzle: Bishop Robinson says rehabilitation is key to fixing correctional system," *Baltimore Evening Sun*, August 21, 1989.

Notice of Infraction or Incident

Appendix to DCR 105-2

Institution _____

I. Name _____ No. _____ Date of Infraction _____ Time _____ A.M. P.M.

A report has been filed charging you with the following violation(s):

Rule # _____ State Facts (What Happened): _____
(See reverse side for explanation of Rule #)

_____

_____

_____

_____

_____

Reporting Officer _____

The report, as stated, has been reviewed by the Shift Commander and the following action has been taken:

☐ Admin. Seg.   ☐ Refer to Hearing Officer   ☐ Incident Report   ☐ Informal Disposition (State Disposition)

Reason for action taken: _____

Shift Commander's Signature _____ Date _____ Time _____ A.M. P.M.

Notified of Incident Report: ☐ Yes   ☐ No   I accept Informal Disposition   ☐ Yes   ☐ No

Inmate's Signature _____ Number _____ Date _____

II. **SERVICE NOTICE**   NOTE: Failure to indicate a wish to have representation or witnesses below will be deemed a waiver of the right to representation or witnesses.

Served by _____ Title _____ Date _____ Time _____ A.M. P.M.

In acknowledgement of the charge(s) presented: ☐ I do not want to be represented.   ☐ I do want to be represented, and request

the following person: _____   ☐ I do not want witnesses.   ☐ I do want witnesses, and

request the following persons: _____

NOTE: If you are currently on probation by virtue of a previous adjustment violation, please be aware that your probation may be revoked by committing another offense and all sanctions deferred as a result of that probation may be added to those received, if you are found guilty of the current offense(s).

Name _____ Number _____ Date _____

III. **WAIVER OF 24-HOUR NOTICE**

I understand that I must be given 24-hour notice before an adjustment hearing in order to prepare my case. I may waive this requirement by signing this section;

Inmate's Signature _____ Date _____

SEE BACK FOR RIGHTS AT HEARING & RIGHTS OF APPEAL

Prepare in duplicate
DC Form 105-2a (Rev. 9/88)

Distribution - Original, Base File
Copy, Inmate

RIGHTS AT HEARING

Refusal to appear before the Hearing Officer constitutes a waiver of the right to a hearing and the Hearing Officer will hear the case in absentia. At the Adjustment Hearing, you have the right to have representation. You may request to have an inmate or employee of the Institution to act as your representative. You will also have the opportunity to call one or more witnesses, if the Hearing Officer determines it to be practical or relevant to your case. Such witnesses may include an accuser and the employee who presented the charges. The Hearing Officer shall allow you to question any witnesses who testify at the hearing, if they deem it to be relevant to your case. At the Adjustment Hearing, you do not have to testify in your own defense. Refusal to testify is not an admission of guilt. Your rights shall not be unreasonably withheld or restricted by the Hearing Officer.

RIGHTS OF APPEAL

Following the Adjustment Hearing, if you object to the Hearing Officer's decision, you have the right to appeal:

1. To the Warden of your institution within five (5) days;
2. The Inmate Grievance Commission within one (1) year;
3. To the Courts.

RULES

CATEGORY I:

Rule # 1. Wrongful killing, assault, battery, or fighting.

Rule # 2. Committing, performing or being involved in any sexual act without consent.

Rule # 3. Inciting, creating, participating in, being involved in any manner, or committing any mutinous act, riot, or disturbance.

Rule # 4. Making or possession of any weapon or any other article which has been modified into a weapon.

Rule # 5. Being involved in any manner with an act of arson or possession of any unauthorized incendiary materials.

Rule # 6. Escape.

CATEGORY II:

Rule # 7. Setting a fire or sounding a false alarm.

Rule # 8. Being involved in any manner with a consensual sexual act.

Rule # 9. Possession of any implements which could reasonably be used to perpetrate an escape.

Rule #10. Any act of extortion, coersion or bribery.

Rule #11. Violation of any specifically cited federal, state or local statute, law, or ordinance not otherwise included in these regulations.

Rule #12. Violation of any specifically cited rule or regulation applicable to any special program; e.g., work release, authorized leave, etc.

Rule #13. Use, possession without authorization, or distribution of any substance which could reasonably be used as an intoxicant, any controlled dangerous substance as defined in Art. 27 of the Annotated Code of Maryland, or any paraphernalia used to administer the same as defined by Maryland law.

Rule #14. Use, possession, distribution, or accumulating unauthorized medication, hoarding or accumulating authorized medication, or the use or possession of quinine in any form.

Rule #15. Stealing or possession of stolen property.

Rule #16. Refusal to submit to any lawful and properly authorized test for detection of drugs or alcohol.

Rule #17. Possession of money (coin or paper), checks, or money orders without authorization or in excess of the amount authorized by the rules of the institution or unit in which one is housed.

CATEGORY III:

Rule #18. Possession of, passing, or receiving contraband, regardless of the place of occurrence. Contraband is any article which an inmate is not permitted to trade, loan, give away, or possess by Division of Correction Regulations or by the rules of the institution or unit in which one is housed.

Rule #19. Leaving from, or being late or absent from, any assigned area without permission; or being in any unassigned or otherwise unauthorized area without permission.

Rule #20. Forgery, alteration, or misrepresentation of any paper, document, or identification badge or possession of same.

Rule #21. Knowingly or intentionally giving anyone false information relating to institutional matters

Rule #22. Performing personal services for any staff member.

Rule #23. Disobeying any direct lawful order given by any staff member.

Rule #24. Refusal to work, accept housing, or carry out an institutional assignment.

Rule #25. Resisting or interfering with the performance of the lawful duties of any staff member.

Rule #26. Destruction, alteration, defacing, tampering with, or misusing any property, equipment, material, tools, or machinery belonging to another.

Rule #27. Exhibition, demonstration, or conveyance of vulgarity, insolence, threat, or disrespect, in any manner, toward any person.

Rule #28. Refusal to be searched or have possessions or quarters searched.

CATEGORY IV:

Rule #30. Failure to possess or display an authorized Division of Correction identification badge.

Rule #31. Stealing, receiving giving away or possessing unauthorized food.

Rule #32. Engaging in horseplay or otherwise behaving in a reckless or negligent manner.

Rule #33. Gambling or possession of gambling paraphernalia.

Rule #34. Unauthorized use of any telephone.

Rule #35. Failure to maintain personal cleanliness, or cleanliness or good order in one's housing area or cell.

Rule #36. Violation of any specifically cited institutional rule which has the approval of the managing officer, yet which is not included in this regulation.

were notified that help might be needed. A video camera was set up on the hospital roof to record suspicious movements in the yard. Experienced guards were assigned to the various posts, and on Tuesday, July 16, the eight-to-four day-shift was told that something might happen.[29]

In C dormitory during the 8:45 P.M. lock-in, Corporal Larry Hughes discovered several hacksaw blades hidden on tier 3 and turned them over to Corporal Cornell Barnes down at the guard desk. Back on the third tier, Hughes was relieved of his keys at gunpoint by two masked inmates and locked in a cell. Minutes later, ringleader Clarence Mouzone held a gun on Barnes at the guard desk, retrieved the hacksaw blades, and ordered him to open the gate for three incoming correctional officers, all of whom were handcuffed and placed in a cell. Mouzone then learned from inmates trying to open a trap door in the dormitory ceiling that it was welded shut. Realizing their situation was hopeless, Mouzone surrendered himself to the guards in the cell and was led out of C dormitory to waiting officers.

The escape attempt having failed, riotous inmates rampaged through the cellblock, setting fires and trashing cells. They robbed, raped, and assaulted other inmates who did not wish to join the rebellion. Officer Hughes was blindfolded and taken up to a fifth tier cell, where he was later joined by another hostage, Corporal Gary Wooten.

Shortly after midnight, heavily armed area tactical units began to arrive, as well as a negotiating team that included Warden Sewall Smith and Commissioner of Corrections Richard Lanham. The negotiation team worked throughout the night and the next morning, when they were joined by inmate Dennis Wise, president of the Inmate Advisory Council,[30] who helped them arrange the release of Officer Wooten shortly before noon. The rebellious inmates told officials they would hold the remaining hostage, Officer Hughes, until they could present their grievances—mainly about overcrowding and food service—to the press. At 3:30 P.M., reporters and television newsmen were escorted into yard #4, where inmate Wise relayed messages from those inside C dormitory. They refused to release hostage Hughes, their last bargaining chip, until they received guarantees that they would not be beaten in retaliation.

The tense stand-off continued, with a state police helicopter hovering over-

---

[29]The account of this riot is based on penitentiary files and newspaper articles: "Pen inmates free officers, end takeover," *Baltimore Sun*, July 18, 1991, and "The Power of the Pen," *Baltimore Sun Magazine*, July 5, 1992.

[30]The Inmate Advisory Council mediated between the prisoners and prison officials. The leader was voted into his position annually ("Pen returning to normal after inmate food boycott," *Baltimore Evening Sun*, February 28, 1989). Wise was also leader of one of the two Islamic groups in the prison and requested the help of the other leader during the negotiations ("The Power of the Pen," *Baltimore Sun Magazine*, July 5, 1992).

head, attack dogs straining at their leashes, and SWAT team members positioned along the wall. Time was running out. Taking a chance, Warden Smith walked alone into C dormitory and finally arranged for the release of the last hostage at 8 P.M. Thanks to patient negotiating and the use of an influential inmate go-between, prison officials had been able to defuse an explosive situation. No prisoners were beaten in retaliation, but thirty-four of them were placed in segregation as a result of the hostage-taking incident.

Then, late in 1991, occurred an escape as daring and sensational in its own way as that of "Tunnel Joe" Holmes forty years earlier. On a Saturday afternoon, November 30, a guard at Supermax across Madison Street from the penitentiary noticed bits of clothing caught in the razor wire near the cell windows on the top floor. It was the trail of convicted murderer Harry Benjamin Dean, 40, the first inmate to escape from one of the most technologically advanced, supposedly escape-proof prisons built in this country.[31]

Dean, serving life plus 105 years, had managed to squeeze his slender frame (five feet, eleven inches, 145 pounds) through the narrow cell window (six inches high and fourteen inches wide, which he enlarged to eight by twenty-two inches), hoist himself up about twelve feet to the roof with a makeshift rope of clothing and grappling hook, and lower himself down to Constitution Street. Blood found on the rooftop indicated he might have cut himself severely on the razor wire while fleeing.

A combination of structural weakness in the prison and lax security by the guards made possible his escape. Instead of being handcuffed and escorted to his shower by two officers as called for by the rules, his cell door was opened remotely from the control booth. He declined the shower, dropped out of view of the video cameras, and crawled into the next cell, whose occupant, John Dempsey, had also declined the shower and was waiting. Using a makeshift screwdriver fashioned by Dean from a piece of metal from his orthopedic shoes (he had broken his ankle during a previous escape from the penitentiary), the two inmates opened the security screen covering the window and used smuggled saw blades to cut the outer window. Dempsey could not squeeze through the narrow opening, but Dean could—and did. He was apprehended by the FBI ten months later in Ohio.[32] An "unclimbable" chain link fence was subsequently installed surrounding the roof to block future escapes by that route.[33]

By now, the penitentiary's notorious south wing was being phased out.

---

[31]"Killer makes first escape at 'Supermax,'" *Baltimore Sun,* December 1, 1991; "Escape raises security issues at 'Supermax,'" *Baltimore Sun,* December 2, 1991; and "'Supermax' escape foiled the latest in prison technology," *Baltimore Sun,* December 8, 1991.

[32]"FBI finds killer in Ohio town," *Baltimore Sun,* October 9, 1992.

[33]"Only one to escape Supermax prison given 5 more years," *Baltimore Sun,* March 27, 1993.

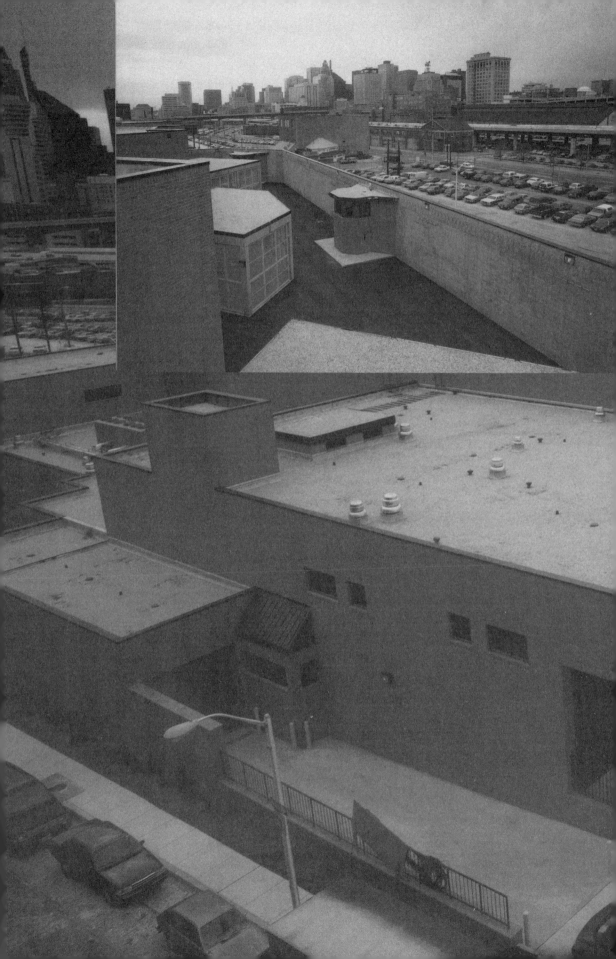

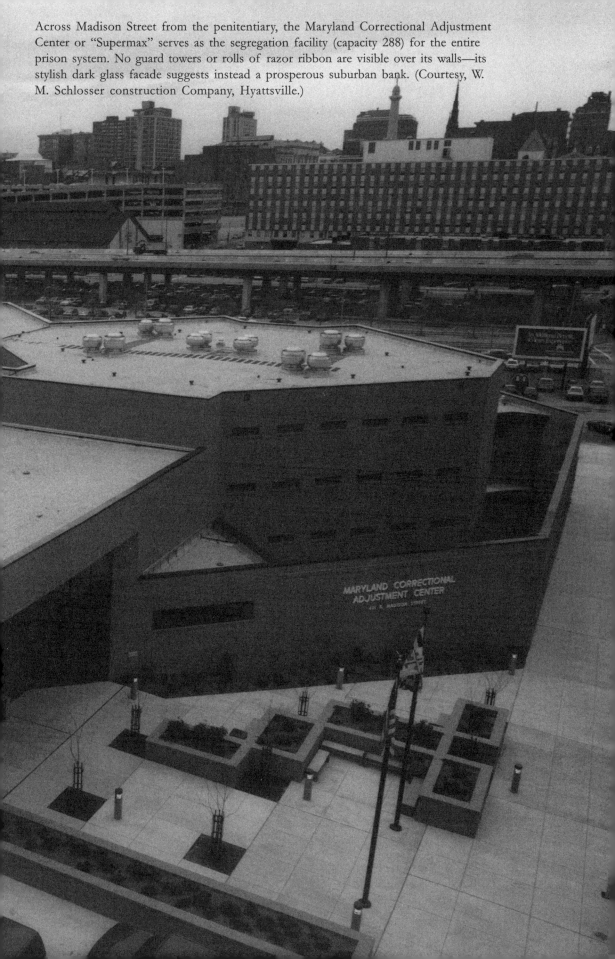

Across Madison Street from the penitentiary, the Maryland Correctional Adjustment Center or "Supermax" serves as the segregation facility (capacity 288) for the entire prison system. No guard towers or rolls of razor ribbon are visible over its walls—its stylish dark glass facade suggests instead a prosperous suburban bank. (Courtesy, W. M. Schlosser construction Company, Hyattsville.)

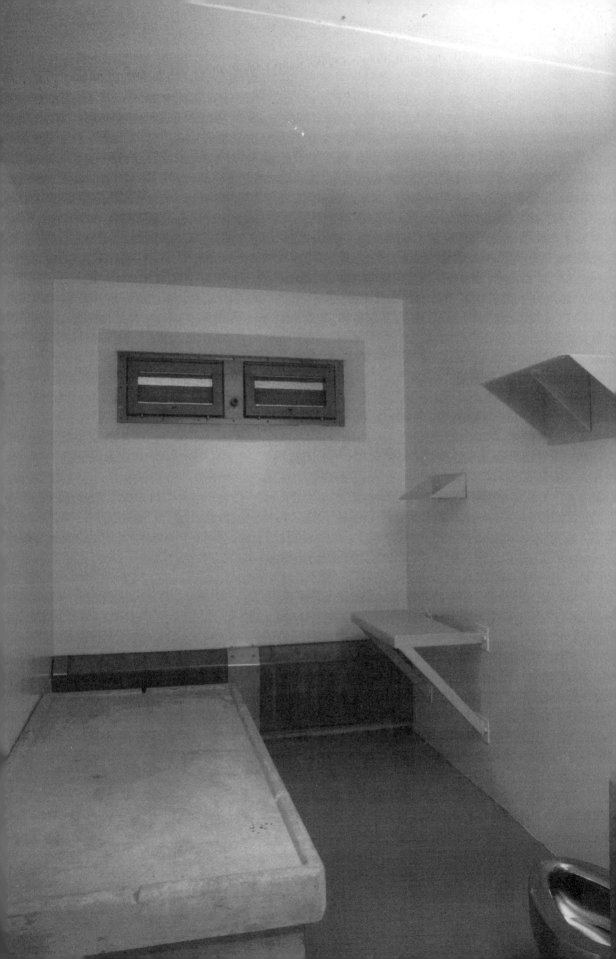

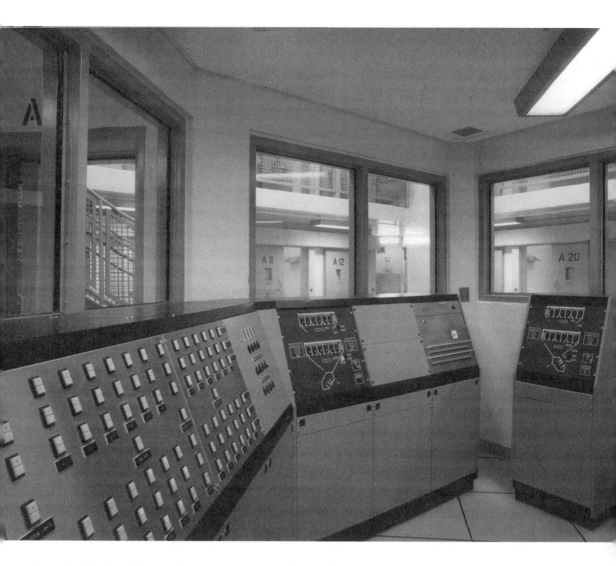

Opposite: Designed for maximum security, this concrete cell has a concrete slab bed—to be covered with a flame-resistant mattress—that cannot be broken apart to make weapons. The window was made narrow, fourteen inches wide and six inches high, to prevent the inmate from wriggling through. But on November 30, 1991, Harold Benjamin Dean widened the slot by unscrewing the metal casement and squeezed his way to freedom. The cell windows have since been modified to prevent a recurrence.

Above: From this central control booth inside one of three octagonal cellhouses of Supermax, one correctional officer can supervise forty-eight surrounding cells and operate the cell doors with the control panel. The circular design is more efficient than rectangular cellblocks, which require more personnel to supervise straight rows of cells. (Photographs courtesy W. M. Schlosser Construction Company.)

Despite temporary repairs, the decrepit five-story steel cellblock standing free within its granite walls had begun to twist and bend under its own weight, necessitating the closing of the cells on its upper tiers. On December 10, 1991, the last thirteen inmates on the ground floor were transferred, and the south wing was empty for the first time in its ninety-two years. After much debate, the state decided to tear down the still serviceable granite shell and build a completely new minimum-security prison on the site, the Metropolitan Transition Services Center, favored by public safety chief Robinson as a means to prepare soon-to-be released inmates for their reentry into society.[34]

For other inmates—those sentenced to death and who had so far managed to evade the final stroke—the skies clouded. Events unfolded that would lead to the penitentiary's first execution in nearly thirty-three years.

Ever since the 1960s, support for capital punishment from a crime-weary public had been steadily growing across the nation. After the Supreme Court reinstated the death penalty in 1976, Maryland followed suit in 1978 but did not act on it for the next sixteen years. Then somewhat reluctantly, it became the twenty-third state to resume executions. In March 1994, Maryland adopted as its primary method lethal injection, first used by Texas in 1982 and generally regarded as more humane than all other methods of execution.[35]

Three-time killer John Thanos, 45, had refused to appeal his death sentence and even protested filings on his behalf by the federal public defenders' office in Baltimore and the American Civil Liberties Union. Early on the morning of May 17, 1994, he was strapped down on a steel table next to the old gas chamber in the penitentiary hospital. Asked at the very last minute if he wanted to halt his execution and initiate the appeals process, he replied, "Let's get on with it." He died quietly, without outward sign of suffering. But condemned inmates at the penitentiary now realized that any one of them could be next.[36]

The year 1995 brought with it two major changes that together ended the Maryland Penitentiary's historic role as the state's only maximum-security prison. First, on July 12, the four-hundred-bed minimum-security Metropolitan Transition Services Center[37] opened on the site of the penitentiary's old south wing. Like its predecessor, this facility is rectangular but is designed for more effi-

---

[34]"'Circle of hell,' Pen's South Wing, holds tormented souls no longer," *Baltimore Sun,* December 18, 1991, and "Razing of prison is faulted," *Baltimore Sun,* March 9, 1993.

[35]"The Death Penalty Myth," *Baltimore Sunday Sun,* June 5, 1988; "Lethal Injection," *Washington Post Health Supplement,* December 11, 1990, pp. 13–15; "State Ready to Give Thanos Lethal Injection," *Baltimore Sun,* May 6, 1994; "Lethal-injection Table Ready for Thanos," *Baltimore Sun,* May 8, 1994; and "Execution Puts Md. With 22 Other States," *Baltimore Sun,* May 18, 1994.

[36]"Thanos Died Quietly After a Life of Fury," *Baltimore Sun,* May 18, 1994.

[37]Designed by Architectural Technologies and built by Cam Construction Company at a cost of $13 million.

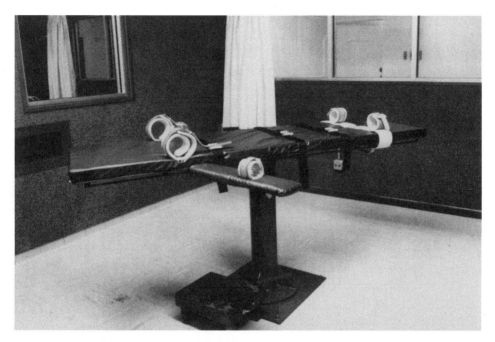

In 1994 yet another change was made in the method of execution. The condemned prisoner is strapped onto a table and given a lethal injection of drugs, which first puts the person to sleep, then paralyzes the breathing muscles, and finally stops the heart. (Courtesy, Lt. James Felix.)

cient, safer surveillance and control of its inmates. Instead of the old straight-line tiers of cells fronted by catwalks, it has four, fifty-bed dormitories at the corners of its two floors. On each floor, a centrally located control booth—shaped somewhat like a trolley car—allows the officer at each end to monitor two dormitories at once on TV screens and operate the doors from within electronically. The facility has its own entrance, and its inmates reach the penitentiary's cafeteria by a route separate from that used by higher-risk penitentiary inmates, with whom they are not allowed to mix.

The minimum-security inmates at MTSC are typically short-timers, having one to eighteen months left to serve before being released. Case management workers meet with them to determine which program will best prepare them for reentry into society: boot camp (generally for young, non-violent offenders); home detention (with electronic monitoring); job training at the Occupational Skills Training Center across Forrest Street; or residence in the local Dismas House (a traditional half-way house). These programs are voluntary: inmates have to sign up but get credit toward release.[38]

---

[38]The description of MTSC in these two paragraphs is based on a tour of the facility on September 14, 1995, and interviews with Administrator Lehrman W. Dotson and caseworkers Mark Waranch and Chevette Henson.

The other major change at the penitentiary in 1995 began in July and took a year to complete. Gradually, the maximum-security inmates in the general population were transferred in van loads to the House of Correction Annex in Jessup, a recently built (opened 1991) maximum-security facility with a more efficient design. Their beds at the penitentiary were to be filled by medium-security inmates brought in from the whole prison system.[39] The penitentiary's obsolete dormitories—once the pride of the city and state—will continue to house the less dangerous offenders until renovated or replaced entirely.

The removal of its more dangerous prisoners should help penitentiary officials keep the lid on its swarm of sometimes unruly inmates and make it a safer place for inmates and correctional officers alike. But pressure from overcrowding will continue in prisons across the nation since the passage of tougher sentencing laws, such as the so-called "three-strikes" law (life sentences for three-time felony offenders) passed early in 1994.[40] With the exception of Supermax, whose number of inmates has recently decreased,[41] the penitentiary shares the problem of overcrowding with other facilities in Maryland's prison system (23,000 inmates, 14,000 capacity). Though the growth rate of inmates has slowed somewhat in Maryland and across the nation for the past three years, from 1993 through 1995,[42] many observers fear this abatement is the lull before a storm of crime and violence from a baby boom "echo" of young offenders.

Even with the penitentiary's changeover to a medium-security prison, its administrators will continue to face another kind of pressure—that of public opinion. The news media will be there, as always, waiting for a sensational story, be it a riot, escape, suicide, rape or murder. Moreover, inmates can now generate unfavorable publicity by filing complaints with such bodies as the State Grievance Commission, the Legal Aid Bureau of Prisoner Assistance Project, the Maryland State Bar Association, and the Maryland Commission for Responsible Corrections Policy.[43] Satisfying the public is also more difficult for prison officials everywhere. Changes in political and economic conditions and in the crime rate cause the public mood to swing between the conservative warehouse mentality ("lock 'em up and throw the key away") and the liberal emphasis on short prison sentences, rehabilitation programs, and extensive use of parole.

---

[39]Interview with the penitentiary's audit coordinator, Andrew Stritch, January 22, 1996.

[40]"U.S. goes on binge of prison building," *Baltimore Sun,* May 9, 1994, and "Longer state sentences urged," *Baltimore Sun,* April 7, 1995.

[41]"Tough prison cuts number of inmates," *Baltimore Sun,* December 28, 1995.

[42]"Crime figures drop for 3rd straight year," *Baltimore Sun,* May 22, 1995, and "Down goes the crime rate — why?" *Baltimore Sun,* January 15, 1996.

[43]Recently, however, abuses of this privilege by inmates have led to restrictions by federal and state officials. See "Justices do about-face on inmate rights," *Baltimore Sun,* June 20, 1995, and "Curran, other state attorneys general push to curb inmate suits," *Baltimore Sun,* August 2, 1995.

However, as this essay has tried to show, administrators of the Maryland Penitentiary have almost always responded positively over the years to public opinion as well as to new ideas in prison architecture and penology. But their good intentions were subject to the technology and funding available, political cross-currents, and the limitations of human nature itself in both the prisoners and their keepers. The penitentiary's very beginning as an institution in 1804 arose from the public's desire to abolish the spectacle of convicts working in wheelbarrow gangs on the streets of Baltimore Town and remove them to a secluded place where they could reform themselves through productive labor. When the congregate nightrooms of the first prison dormitory (1811) proved unsatisfactory because they offered opportunities for "evil association" (moral contamination), officials chose for their second dormitory (1829) the new, cost-efficient Auburn design to house convicts at night in monastic isolation. When the numerous workshops scattered throughout the prison proved too difficult to supervise properly, a central workshop complex was constructed (1836) using an innovative radial plan that allowed closer surveillance with fewer guards and that increased productivity of the prisoners.

When in 1836–37 the weavers of Baltimore accused the penitentiary of unfair competition, penitentiary officials—despite a bitter personal feud being carried on amongst them at the time—united to defend successfully the young institution during a full-scale investigation into its affairs by a state legislative committee. The investigation also resulted in a self-cleansing brought about by the penitentiary administration's reform faction, resulting in a streamlined, more efficient administration and the purge of the warden and his cronies for improper conduct.

Over the next half-century, penitentiary officials experimented with innovative practices from other prisons and fresh ideas from prison reformers. They substituted the cold shower bath and reduced diet for the standard punishment of whipping, confined juvenile and petty offenders apart from hardened criminals, formed a relief association to help newly discharged convicts reenter society and find jobs, passed a commutation law that allowed time off for good behavior, and permitted prisoners such privileges as exercise, use of a library, and holiday entertainments to reduce the boredom of their lives. Toward the end of the 1880s, the notably reform-minded Warden John W. Horn called for the expansion of the prison northward and construction of a wholly modern prison, but the state legislature would not vote for the necessary funds.

A break in the penitentiary's progressivism occurred during the years of Warden John F. Weyler's autocratic reign (1888–1912). Weyler drove his convict laborers to produce ever larger surpluses for the state treasury without heed to their rehabilitation, but even here one could argue that he thought he was giving the public what it wanted: a prison that cost the taxpayers nothing to operate. And undeniably he did push through the construction of a modern granite and steel prison with the latest amenities. The public disclosure of Weyler's despotic regime led to the creation of a state prison board to oversee the penitentiary. His successor, John F. Leonard, moved swiftly to ease prison discipline and emphasize rehabilitation.

The limitations of Warden Leonard's reforms surfaced immediately after his death in 1920, when prisoners staged the worst riot in penitentiary history to test the new administration. Thereafter they repaid the liberal policies of Warden Claude B. Sweezey with a rash of escapes or escape attempts that brought about his resignation in 1925. His successor, Patrick J. Brady, quickly restored order and with his self-described "firm but humane" system of handling convicts steered the penitentiary on a steady and relatively uneventful course for the next twenty-two years through the conservative climate of the Depression and World War II. The next warden, Edwin T. Swenson, tightened discipline somewhat but placed more emphasis on rehabilitation, providing facilities for vocational training and hiring the penitentiary's first full-time psychologist to serve the needs of the work and education programs. He was succeeded in 1953 by Vernon L. Pepersack, a man described as "100 percent more lenient," and with an academic background in psychology, sociology, criminology, and social psychology. His management more clearly reflected the newly revived penal philosophy that viewed prisoners as mental patients who needed psychological treatment, education, and vocational training to enable them to reenter society. Most of his tenure proved quiet too, partly because the social and political conformity of the Eisenhower era discouraged disruptive behavior. It proved to be the calm before the storm.

The early 1960s ushered in the climactic phase of the Civil Rights Movement in 1963, led by Martin Luther King Jr., which tended to politicize black inmates at the penitentiary. The next year saw the beginning of the anti-Vietnam War movement, whose highly publicized demonstrations and riots further encouraged inmates—black and white alike—to take direct action for their own grievances. The elevation that same year of the penitentiary's easy-going Warden Pepersack to the post of commissioner of corrections tended to weaken discipline among guards and prisoners throughout the entire system and—along with the two outside political movements—helped produce the prison system's first serious riots in many years. The resulting investigations by the state police, Maryland's attorney general, and the Michaelson Commission brought swift corrective measures, including Pepersack's dismissal.

Thereafter, until 1980, the turmoil within the prison system continued as liberal policies and experiments initiated at a higher level clashed with the conservative mindset of veteran line officers, many of whom resigned. The Maryland Penitentiary alone saw an unprecedented turnover of five wardens from 1964 to 1974. Toward the end of the 1970s, crime and violence on the streets increased exponentially. The crisis was due mainly to the epidemic drug culture and the resultant decline of tightly knit neighborhoods and the family unit (graphically described in West Baltimore by David Simon in his documentary book *Homicide: A Year on the Killing Streets,* 1991). Shifting social and moral values evoked a nationwide call to "get tough" with criminals. An influx of drug offenders caused prisons to become dangerously overcrowded. In Maryland, the tangible result was an expensive ten-year prison construction program, during which the penitentiary's facilities were renovated and enlarged. An early release program—greater use of probation, half-way houses, and parole—was tried to ease the crisis. The abuses by inmates of this program resulted in a public backlash and the call for sterner measures.

At this writing, the public mood in Maryland remains conservative and punitive, calling for tougher sentences for violent offenders and no parole for lifers. If and when that mood swings back to a liberal emphasis on expensive educational and job-training programs to rehabilitate inmates for their eventual release, Maryland Penitentiary administrators will doubtless do what they have almost always done throughout its long history: give the public what it wants—and is willing to pay for.

In the always imperfect world of correctional institutions, the Maryland Penitentiary has left behind an honorable record over nearly two centuries. Its castle-like administration building still stands at the corner of Eager and Forrest Streets as a monument to the good intentions of the state.

Appendix A

Wardens of the Maryland Penitentiary

Edward Markland	December 31, 1811	to	April 18, 1812
Nathaniel Hynson	April 18, 1812	to	February 23, 1814
Benjamin Williams	February 23, 1814	to	March 14, 1821
Nathaniel Hynson	March 14, 1821	to	February 9, 1825
Joseph Owens	February 9, 1825	to	March 1839
William Houlton	March 1839	to	March 19, 1842
A. I. W. Jackson	March 19, 1842	to	February 17, 1845
William Johnson	February 17, 1845	to	March 16, 1848
Isaac M. Denson	March 16, 1848	to	June 19, 1851
William H. Jenkins	June 19, 1851	to	March 15, 1852
O. P. Merryman	March 15, 1852	to	June 1858
A. D. Evans	June 1858	to	May 15, 1862
Mark C. W. Thompson	May 15, 1862	to	May 16, 1867
John W. Horn	May 16, 1867	to	May 15, 1872
Thomas S. Wilkinson	May 15, 1872	to	March 2, 1882
John W. Horn	May 4, 1882	to	May 30, 1888
John F. Weyler	June 1, 1888	to	May 1, 1912
John F. Leonard	May 1, 1912	to	August 5, 1920
Claude B. Sweezey	October 1, 1920	to	May 31, 1925
Patrick J. Brady	June 1, 1925	to	July 1, 1947
Edwin T. Swenson	September 1, 1947	to	April 12, 1953
Vernon L. Pepersack	May 8, 1953	to	April 21, 1964
Franklin K. Brough	May 20, 1964	to	March 11, 1966
Roger B. Copinger	June 1, 1966	to	October 23, 1968
Preston L. Fitzberger	October 16, 1968	to	March 16, 1971
Leonard L. Decker	October 13, 1971	to	July 31, 1972
Gerald H. McClellan	July 5, 1972	to	March 1974
George Collins	October 9, 1974	to	October 18, 1983
Leslie H. Dorsey	October 19, 1983	to	November 14, 1984
Howard N. Lyles	November 15, 1984	to	December 31, 1987
James N. Rollins	January 19, 1988	to	March 14, 1991
Sewall B. Smith	July 1, 1991	to	June 30, 1994
Eugene M. Nuth	July 1, 1994		

Appendix B

Executions at the Maryland Penitentiary

By Hanging

1.	Bl	21	George Shelton	Rape	June 8, 1923
2.	Bl	18	Carroll Gibson	Rape	February 13, 1925
3.	Bl	37	Isaac Benson	Murder	July 23, 1926
4.	Wh	27	Richard Reese Whittemore	Murder	August 13, 1926
5.	Bl	19	Ottie Simmons	Murder	September 9, 1927
6.	Bl	20	Arthur Swann	Murder	September 9, 1927
7.	Bl	23	William Henry Rose	Murder	September 9, 1927
8.	Bl	19	Alfred Simms	Rape	November 11, 1927
9.	Wh	28	Benjamin F. Spragins	Murder	August 3, 1928
10.	Wh	28	Charles P. Carey	Murder	August 3, 1928
11.	Bl	27	Hopkins Watkins	Murder	November 16, 1928
12.	Wh	51	John Orestus Marsh	Murder	August 9, 1929
13.	Bl	55	John Jackson	Murder	January 31, 1930
14.	Bl	32	Lorenzo Price	Murder	June 12, 1931
15.	Bl	42	Thomas Blackson	Murder	January 15, 1932
16.	Bl	28	Walter F. Wright	Murder	April 8, 1932
17.	Bl	60	Buel Lee	Murder	October 27, 1933
18.	Bl	46	Page Jupiter	Murder	February 2, 1934
19.	Bl	30	Gordon Dent	Murder	April 19, 1935
20.	Bl	25	James A. Cross	Murder	April 19, 1935
21.	Bl	45	William Harold	Rape	June 28, 1935
22.	Bl	27	James Poindixter	Rape	June 28, 1935
23.	Wh	22	Augusto Perez	Rape	June 12, 1936
24.	Bl	25	Willie Williams	Murder	June 12, 1936
25.	Bl	20	James Irvin Howard	Murder	July 9, 1937
26.	Bl	31	Richard Hammond	Murder	August 28, 1938
27.	Bl	25	James Albert Turner	Rape	August 29, 1938
28.	Wh	44	Fred Brown	Murder	March 19, 1939
29.	Wh	40	Thomas C. Sanchez	Rape	March 15, 1940
30.	Wh	23	Alvin Kenton	Rape	March 15, 1940
31.	Bl	28	William T. Sorrell	Murder	May 10, 1940
32.	Bl	23	Otis Harrell	Murder	May 10, 1940
33.	Bl	33	Alexander Williams	Rape	June 28, 1940
34.	Bl	27	Arthur B. Collick	Murder	September 13, 1940
35.	Wh	33	Wilson Knott	Rape	January 10, 1941
36.	Bl	23	French Lee White	Rape	June 27, 1941
37.	Wh	22	Earl Loveless	Murder	September 26, 1941
38.	Wh	29	James Lee Miller	Murder	September 26, 1941
39.	Bl	38	James Baker	Murder	December 19, 1941
40.	Bl	37	Wilber Pritcheet	Rape	May 8, 1942

41.	Bl	32	Frank Haywood	Rape	June 5, 1942
42.	Bl	54	Andrew Henry	Rape	June 5, 1942
43.	Bl	23	Charles J. Benjamin	Murder	July 10, 1942
44.	Bl	27	Edward Woffard	Murder	July 24, 1942
45.	Bl	39	James Gilliam	Murder	July 24, 1942
46.	Bl	32	James Ford	Murder	January 15, 1943
47.	Bl	23	Frank Williams	Rape	March 12, 1943
48.	Bl	21	Freeman Holton	Murder	June 4, 1943
49.	Bl	19	John Lampkin	Murder	June 4, 1943
50.	Bl	33	William Charles Holsey	Rape	August 13, 1943
51.	Bl	20	Martin Smith	Murder	February 25, 1944
52.	Bl	25	John Hinton	Rape	March 31, 1944
53.	Bl	24	Calvin W. Watkins	Rape	June 16, 1944
54.	Wh	40	Patrick Murphy	Murder	November 17, 1944
55.	Bl	28	Luther McClam	Rape	July 20, 1945
56.	Wh	31	Donald Brooks	Murder	August 17, 1945
57.	Bl	38	John Henry Fields	Murder	November 30, 1945
58.	Bl	21	William Tasker	Murder	December 28, 1945
59.	Bl	22	Lloyd Walker	Murder	January 18, 1946
60.	Bl	22	Roy Nathan Peters	Rape	August 9, 1946
61.	Bl	22	William Daniel Demby	Rape	October 4, 1946
62.	Bl	25	Jack Lister Barnes	Rape	October 4, 1946
63.	Bl	19	Charles Lee Carmen	Rape	December 13, 1946
64.	Bl	20	William E. Copper	Rape	January 17, 1947
65.	Bl	18	Weldon Jones Jr.	Rape	June 27, 1947
66.	Wh	24	Ross J. Abbott	Murder	August 1, 1947
67	Bl	22	Ollie Smith Jr.	Murder	August 1, 1947
68.	Bl	32	Henry T. Jackson	Rape	April 30, 1948
69.	Wh	39	Roy Lee Lathco	Murder	April 30, 1948
70.	Wh	31	Howard A. From	Rape	April 30, 1948
71.	Bl	26	John Knowles	Murder	July 8, 1949
72.	Bl	31	Eugene H. James	Murder	August 12, 1949
73.	Bl	31	Lott Glover	Murder	August 25, 1953
74.	Wh	35	George Edward Grammer	Murder	June 11, 1954
75.	Bl	32	William C. Thomas	Murder	June 10, 1955

By Asphyxiation (Gas)

76.	Bl	29	Eddie Lee Daniels	Murder	June 28, 1957
77.	Bl	25	Carl Daniel Kier	Murder	January 21, 1959
78.	Bl	17	Leonard M. Shockey	Murder	April 10, 1959
79.	Bl	33	Nathaniel Lipscomb	Murder	June 9, 1961

The foregoing list was compiled by Watt Espy of the Capital Punishment Research Project (Box 277/100 East Main Street, Headland, Alabama 36345).

By Lethal Injection

80.	Wh	45	John Thanos	Murder	May 17, 1994
81.	Bl	38	Flint Gregory Hunt	Murder	July 2, 1997

Appendix C

Psychology Department

Reprinted from The Courier *(a bimonthly magazine published by inmates of the Maryland Penitentiary), vol. 4, no. 11 (January–February 1961).*

The psychological department's history in this institution, as well as in most institutions, is relatively short, as the field of psychology is one of the newer approaches to the study of penology. To the best of this writer's knowledge there was no formal Psychological Department in the Maryland Penitentiary until this writer came to the institution on April 1, 1948. In looking through old files which date back to the early 1940's, there are occasional reports entitled, "Psycho-pathological reports," by a Dr. Partridge, but there are very few of these reports. Most of the reports give an estimated I.Q. obtained from the old Short Form of the 1916 Stanford Binet Intelligence Scale. They were more of a clinical description of the individual than a psychological evaluation. The institution also had a psychiatrist, who came when called for consultation, and beginning in about 1943 Dr. J. G. N. Cushing came to the institution as a Psychiatric Consultant for one half day each week. From approximately 1944 to 1948 some psychological reports were made by Mr. Charles Lustnaur, who was employed as a teacher within the institution. He also used the Short Form of the Stanford Binet Intelligence Scale referred to above. The reports referred to here usually consisted of a description of the man's behavior and an I.Q. showing the level of his mental capacity.

Perhaps the greatest impetus for establishment of a Psychological Department within the Penitentiary came from Edwin T. Swenson, who became Warden of the Maryland Penitentiary in September of 1947. Through his work as Assistant Warden in the Minnesota State Penitentiary and his subsequent experience as Commandant of the United States Army Disciplinary Barracks at Green Haven, New York, he was well acquainted with the value of a full time Psychological Department in correctional work. This writer [Loyal B. Calkins] worked with Colonel Swenson at the Disciplinary Barracks while in the Army, and it was through Colonel Swenson's friendship that the writer was persuaded to come to the Maryland Penitentiary upon his discharge from the army.

The writer came to the Penitentiary as its first full time psychologist on

April 1, 1948. Colonel Swenson and the writer visualized a psychological program in three phases which are as follows:

Phase I

In 1948 the first step was to get a psychologist to start a psychological program where none existed. The diagnostic need was acute. The need for knowledge of the mental level, personality makeup and problems of the inmates had to be recognized and accomplished. Thus a system of diagnostic tests had to be organized. Before this could be accomplished a psychological survey of the institution had to be made in order to evaluate the psychological problem of the whole institution in its relationship to the individual problems.

To accomplish Phase I every man in the Penitentiary was given a series of group intelligence tests during the year of 1948. These tests were separated into two types, one for the literate and the other for the illiterate inmates. This was accomplished by the end of 1948. In order to have a more accurate idea of the mental level of each inmate, as well as an idea of his more specific talents and abilities, the year 1949 was spent in getting an individual I.Q. examination on each inmate. For this survey the Wechsler Bellevue Intelligence Scale was used. While this was being accomplished we also attempted to get a rough idea of the personality factors of each inmate who was literate by the use of the Minnesota Multiphasic Personality Inventory. By the end of 1949 this project had been accomplished. The writer was aided in this task by Mr. Lustnaur and by two inmates who had been carefully screened and picked from the inmate population. These two inmates were Carl Newman and Alfred Acquilino.

With this accomplishment, the next step of Phase I was to establish a diagnostic organization which would more or less follow an inmate through his development within the institution. Thus an initial testing program was devised for each inmate upon his admission to the Penitentiary. This consisted of both intelligence and personality tests, and a write-up of the evaluation of these tests by the psychologist. These results were presented to the Classification Committee when the inmate appeared for his initial classification. The psychologist was present at these meetings and gave advice as to the inmate's work assignment, security ratings, and housing such as single cell, double cell or dormitory quarters. In 1950 we also organized a plan by which every inmate who was to appear before the Parole Board would be re-evaluated with intelligence tests if it was considered appropriate, but chiefly to be re-evaluated with tests to see if the inmate had been successful in changing his personality during his incarceration. Although intelligence tests give us a good idea of the inmate's capacities for adjustment and achievement, the fact is that people integrate with each other because of their personalities rather than their I.Q.'s. Thus, by the beginning of 1950 Phase I of the program was in operation.

Phase II

The second phase was one of orientation of the psychological program into all aspects of the institution, particularly into the shop and custodial forces. It was only natural that a new department in the institution would be met with some resistance, especially when that department had a duty to make recommendations involving both the shop and custodial programs. This step was accomplished during 1950 and 1951 when the psychologist organized and executed a program of orientation and training of the custodial force, the shop force, and the Classification Department in the psychological approach to inmate problems. This was accomplished by a course of thirteen lectures on the Psychology of Personality as related to this institution, which was given to the above-mentioned departments, including all three custodial shifts. It was both the contention of this writer and Colonel Swenson that the shop officers and custodial officers would respond to such a program although our ideas have been opposed to some authorities in the field. We felt that it was almost impossible for anyone working with people who have problems such as found in an institution of this kind to be uninterested in those problems. It was felt that if they could be given a course in psychological know-how in non-technical terms, and with the emphasis upon practical problems, they would absorb the knowledge and accept the psychological approach. This program was well received by the staff of the institution. The only difficulty in following this program was that the psychologist got many more referrals for examination and treatment of inmates from the personnel of the institution than he could possibly handle.

Phase III

The third phase of the psychological program was that of therapy. Therapy consists of three elements, the first of which are the simple improvements in the environment and facilities offered to the inmate for rehabilitation. Any inmate who has been in this institution over the past ten years certainly has a good idea of the environmental changes and the increase in rehabilitative facilities within the institution. The Psychological Department has had an advisory function in the majority of these changes. There has been a tremendous increase in the educational and recreational facilities of the institution.

By the beginning of 1951 this department was able to put the second step of therapy into operation, in that a few cases were selected for individual counseling on specific problems. However, due to the pressure of routine work, only a few inmates could obtain this type of service. Then in August of 1951 the writer was called back on active duty by the Army for a fifteen month period. During this time Mr. William A. Doyle came to us as a Correctional Psychologist to keep the program going. When the writer returned to the Penitentiary on November 15, 1952, Mr. Doyle was transferred, as Correctional Psychologist, to the Maryland House of Correction. In 1953, this department began its first real attempt at individual treatment, which consisted of a long term psychoanalytically oriented psychotherapy. Unfortunately, the writer could not carry more than three or four such cases and keep up the rest of the workload. Things remained pretty much the same until July of 1957, when we were able to get Mr. Doyle transferred back to the Penitentiary as Correctional Psychologist, which gave the department two psychologists. By September of 1958 we were able to start the first group psychotherapy program in the Penitentiary. (The writer refers the reader to an article in the *Courier* in the spring of 1959.) This group consisted of ten men, and they were in therapy for a little more than eighteen months. Considering the whole population of the institution, this was merely a drop in the bucket, but the program proved successful and it is a fervent hope of this writer that it can be greatly expanded in the future. By October 1959 Mr. Doyle was able to start the second group for group psychotherapy within the institution. By the time this article appears in print the writer will have started the third group in psychotherapy. Group psychotherapy, as well as individual psychotherapy takes between eighteen months and two years and is a long term form of treatment.

Thus, the three phases of the psychological program, which were outlined by the writer and Colonel T. Swenson back in 1948 have been accomplished. However, the hard work of bringing such a program into being really fell upon the shoulders of Warden Vernon L. Pepersack when he became warden in 1953. Had it not been for his cooperation and enthusiastic approval of the program, it could not have been accomplished.

We are now at the stage where we have practically a full realization of Phase I and Phase II of the psychological program and a start on Phase III, which is the phase of both individual and group psychotherapy. Our problem is now to find ways and means by which we can expand the therapy programs so that they will be available to all inmates who desire such treatment. At the present time Mr. Doyle and the writer can only handle three or four cases of individual psychotherapy and one group of ten men for group psychotherapy. It is the expansion of this program which is the future goal of the Psychological Department.

Appendix D

Penitentiary Slang

Some prison slang is universal and enduring, such as *fish* (newly arrived prisoner), *snitch* (informer), *shank* (homemade knife), and *punk* (homosexual, usually passive). But much of it is fleeting. *Duke* refers to state issue tobacco of low quality, named for California Governor Deukmejian. Some slang is peculiar to certain prisons. B*onnaroo* means impeccable grooming or sharp dress, as when prison clothes are starched and pressed, showing that the wearer has influence, and *Jim Jones juice* refers to Kool-aid, used sometimes to deliver medicine to inmates who resist medication. Both are used only at Folsom or San Quentin in California.[1] But enduring or not, prison slang is almost always colorful and full of human interest, revealing much about the daily lives of the people who use it.

Among the most enduring slang expressions used at the Maryland Penitentiary are the following: *peepers* (mirrors held outside cell door bars to monitor movements of guards on tier walkways), *fishing* (the technique used to pass contraband from a cell on one tier to another cell on a tier below, using a string or line made of rags tied together), *correctional cocktail* (used by guards to describe a mixture of urine and feces sometimes thrown at them in a plastic cup by unruly inmates in the segregation unit), and *red tag* (file status for particularly dangerous inmates who must be kept under close custody or surveillance).[2] In the prison population, the *oldheads* are inmates who have served a lot of time and generally are not considered troublesome[3] (a saying at the penitentiary is that "Five percent of the inmates cause ninety-five percent of the trouble."[4]), and the *hoppers* are young inmates, especially those who *buck* (riot or rebel) against the prison administration instead of serving their time quietly.[5]

Rhyming slang can be found in such expressions as *log of fogs* (carton of cigarettes, not only smoked but used as prison currency where money is officially prohibited) and *perk and jerk* (concentrated coffee, made so by being con-

---

[1]"A Convict's Dictionary of Words and Phrases," compiled by James Harris in Morrie Camhie, *The Prison Experience* (Rutland, Vt.: Charles Tuttle, 1989), pp. 28, 31, and 34.

[2]*Report on Security Conditions at Maryland Penitentiary's South Wing* (Baltimore: Attorney General's Office, 1984), p. 43; and interview with Andrew Stritch, Audit Coordinator, Maryland Penitentiary, May 3, 1996.

[3]Parole officer Roger Thompson, 1988.

[4]Classification Supervisor Pamela Sorensen, 1989.

[5]Anonymous inmate letter to Warden James Rollins, 1988.

stantly boiled and replenished). Certain expressions can be made up for the occasion and then used repeatedly, as in the case of a somewhat illiterate, old-time assistant warden at the penitentiary, who combined slang and official jargon when writing up charge sheets on inmates: *eyeballing with attempt to signify* (hostile eye contact from an inmate to any official), and *moping with attempt to creep* (shirking one's assigned work).[6] One purely invented word is *blicky,* a universal noun used for just about anything, be it a book or a vacuum cleaner ("put the blicky over there").[7]

Surely the most enduring and colorful slang expression is *jump steady* or *jump,* the name used at the Maryland Penitentiary for illicit homebrew made from ingredients stolen from the kitchen (potatoes, rice, bread, raisins, citrus fruits, fruit juice or tomato puree and sugar). They are mixed together with water and left to ferment for a few days in any available container (a plastic trash barrel, even a plastic garbage bag placed inside a cardboard box, etc.). One doubtful explanation for the origin of *jump steady* is that it came from a test of reflexes imposed by correctional officers on inmates suspected of drinking it. Suspects were ordered to jump into the air—if they could manage a steady landing, they could avoid being charged with violating the prison rule against alcohol.[8]

A more convincing explanation comes from a long-time Baltimore resident, who dates it from the 1920s, when Prohibition was in force. *Jump steady* originated in the black community as a term for bootleg whiskey and its mood-enhancing effect, as when jazz pianist Fats Waller sang, "This joint is jumping."[9] Thereafter, apparently, it was taken over by penitentiary inmates to designate any homebrew.

A full study of slang used at the Maryland Penitentiary by inmates and correctional officers should be done by someone with the right opportunities and linguistic background. It would be a valuable contribution to the penitentiary's history. As cultural anthropologist Franz Boas said, "Language *is* culture."

---

[6]Warden Eugene Nuth, 1994.

[7]Retired Correctional Officer Thomas Tivvis, 1995.

[8]"Prison Officials Confiscate Illegal Brew," *Baltimore Sun,* December 30, 1989.

[9]Interview March 13, 1996 with eighty-four-year-old Richard Powell, long associated with the Negro Baseball League Baltimore Elite Giants, where Roy Campanella and Junior Gilliam began their careers. Mr. Powell's dating of the phrase from the 1920s is supported by a contemporary poster advertising a revue at the Douglas Theatre, "The Snappy Musical Comedy Sensation, *Jump Steady,*" which was displayed at the Enoch Pratt Free Library on August 15, 1990.

Bibliography

Anyone wishing to do further research into the history of the Maryland Penitentiary for the first hundred years or so of its existence will have to rely heavily on the annual reports of its board of directors because of the scarcity of other published materials. The surviving reports are listed below along with the locations. After 1916, control of the penitentiary passed from its board of directors to the newly created State Board of Prison Control, which published annual reports under its auspices. These reports are widely available, especially at the Maryland Room of the Enoch Pratt Free Library, the State Law Library, and the Division of Correction Headquarters.

EP – Maryland Room, Enoch Pratt Free Library, Baltimore, Maryland
MHS – Maryland Historical Society, Baltimore, Maryland
JHU – Eisenhower Library, The Johns Hopkins University, Baltimore, Maryland
DOC – Maryland Division of Correction Headquarters, Baltimore, Maryland
MSA – Maryland State Archives, Annapolis, Maryland
SLL – State Law Library, Annapolis, Maryland

1817/1818 – EP
1819
1820
1821
1822 – MHS
1823 – MHS
1824
1825 – MHS
1826 – EP
1827
1828 – MHS, EP
1829 – MHS
1830 – MHS
1831 – MHS
1832
1833 – MHS, DOC

1834 – MHS
1835 – MHS
1836 – MHS, EP, DOC
1837 – MHS, EP
1838 – EP
1839 – SLL, DOC
1840 – DOC
1841 – EP, DOC
1842
1843 – MHS, DOC
1844 – MHS, DOC
1845 – MHS, EP
1846 – MHS, EP, DOC
1847 – MHS, EP
1848 – MHS, DOC
1849 – DOC

1850 – SLL

1851

1852 – MHS, SLL, DOC

1853 – MHS, EP, SLL

1854 – SLL

1855

1856 – MHS, DOC

1857

1858 – MHS, EP, SLL

1859 – MHS, EP, SLL, DOC

1860 – SLL

1861 – MHS, EP, SLL, DOC

1862 – MHS, SLL

1863 – MHS, DOC

1864 – EP

1865

1866 – MHS, EP, SLL

1867 – MHS

1868 – SLL

1869 – MHS, SLL

1870 – EP, SLL, DOC

1871 – EP, DOC

1872 – EP, SLL, DOC

1873 – EP, SLL

1874 – MHS, EP, SLL, DOC

1875 – EP

1876 – EP, SLL, DOC

1877 – EP, SLL, DOC

1878 – EP, SLL, DOC

1879 – EP, SLL, DOC

1880 – SLL, DOC

1881 – MHS, SLL

1882 – EP

1883 – EP

1884

1885

1886

1887 – SLL

1888 – MSA (Manuscript only)

1889 – SLL

1890 – DOC

1891 – JHU

1892 – EP, JHU, DOC

1893 – JHU, DOC

1894 – JHU, DOC

1895 – EP, DOC

1896 – EP, SLL

1897 – EP, JHU, SLL, DOC

1898 – EP, SLL, DOC

1899 – EP, JHU, SLL, DOC

1900 – EP, SLL

1901 – JHU

1902 – EP

1903 – EP, JHU

1904 – EP, JHU, DOC

1905 – EP, DOC

1906 – EP, DOC

1907 – EP, JHU, DOC

1908 – EP, JHU

1909 – EP, JHU

1910 – EP

1911 – EP

1912 – EP

1913 – EP

1914 – EP

1915 – EP

1916 – EP

1917 – EP

Unpublished Sources

Reception Records of Maryland Penitentiary, 1811–1893. (MSA)

Reception Register of Maryland Penitentiary, 1900–1907. (MSA)

Reception-Discharge Book, Maryland Penitentiary, April 19, 1906–August 1, 1919. (Warden's office)

Prisoners Record, Maryland Penitentiary, January 15, 1919–November 6, 1930. (Warden's office)

Prisoners Record, Maryland Penitentiary, November 6, 1930–October 13, 1943. (Warden's office)

Prisoners Record, Maryland Penitentiary, October 14, 1943–February 18, 1957. (Warden's office)

Return [census] of Prisoners, Maryland Penitentiary, December 1, 1878–November 30, 1913. (Warden's office)

Maryland Penitentiary Index [of all prisoners received], 1812–1948. (Warden's office)

Punishment Book, February 16, 1863–December 29, 1873. (DOC)

Rules Violation Records—Females, 1873–1889. (MSA)

Rules Violations Records, 1873–1909. (DOC)

Violation of Rules, November 9, 1907–May 2, 1912. (DOC)

Punishment Book, February 9, 1920–September 15, 1933. (Warden's office)

Description Book [of inmates, physically], December 1, 1873–November 30, 1878 (DOC)

Description Book, July 25, 1890–December 29, 1899. (DOC)

Letter Book, October 4–December 18, 1909. (DOC)

Bids on Supplies, January 1914–July 1918. (DOC)

Typescripts

Blondo, Richard A. "Samuel Green: A Black Life in Antebellum Maryland." M.A. thesis, University of Maryland, 1988.

Inskeep, Paul (Maryland Penitentiary, #211-806). "A Penitentiary for the Free State." Maryland Penitentiary, 1995.

O'Dunwe, Eugene. "Mr. Jurisprudence." Autobiography, 1938. Owned by his son, David O'Dunne, of Blue Ridge Summit, Pennsylvania.

"Stenographic Record of Testimony Commission Maryland Penitentiary Penal System," Vol. 1. Enoch Pratt Free Library.

Interviews

Interviews cited in this work are not listed here but will be found in the footnotes.

Newspapers

Apart from microfilm, the researcher can consult collections of newspaper articles on the penitentiary (mostly the *Baltimore Sun,* some *Baltimore News-American*) in the vertical files of the Maryland Room at the Enoch Pratt Free Library and in the scrapbooks kept at Maryland Division of Correction headquarters covering the years from 1920 until the 1980s, when systematic computer indexing of *Sun* articles was initiated at the Enoch Pratt Free Library's Maryland Room, and thereafter archived on CD-ROM disks. Individual newspaper articles cited in this work are not listed again here but will be found in the footnotes.

Published Sources

The Acts of Assembly, together with the governor's proclamation and the rules and regulations, respecting the penitentiary of Maryland. Baltimore, 1819.

Andrews, Matthew Page. *Tercentenary History of Maryland.* 4 vols. Baltimore: S. J. Clarke Publishing Co., 1925.

Baltimore City Directory. 1867–68, 1868–69, 1871, 1872, 1873, 1874, 1880, 1887, 1880, 1912, 1913, 1914.

Barnes, Harry Elmer, and Negley K. Teeters. *New Horizons in Criminology.* 3rd edition. Englewood Cliffs, N.J.: Prentice Hall, Inc., 1959.

Bender, John B. *Imagining the Penitentiary: Fictions and the Architecture of Mind in Eighteenth-Century England.* Chicago: University of Chicago Press, 1987.

The Biographical Cyclopedia of Representative Men of Maryland and the District of Columbia. Baltimore: National Biographical Publishing Co., 1879.

Brooks, Neal A., and Richard Parsons. *Baltimore County Panorama.* Towson, Md.: Baltimore County Public Library, 1988.

Brugger, Robert J. *Maryland: A Middle Temperament, 1634–1980.* Baltimore, Md.: The Johns Hopkins University Press, 1988.

Caldwell, Robert. *Red Hannah: Delaware's Whipping Post.* Philadelphia: University of Pennsylvania Press, 1947.

Crawford, William. *Report on the Penitentiaries of the U.S.* 1835. Reprinted Montclair, N.J.: Patterson Smith, 1969.

Crooks, James B. *Politics & Progress: The Rise of Urban Progressivism in Baltimore, 1895–1911.* Baton Rouge: Louisiana State University Press, 1968.

Demetz, M., and Abel Blouet. *Rapport à Monsieur le Comte de Montalivet sur les pénitenciers des États-Unis.* Paris: Imprimerie Royale, 1837.

Depositions taken at the Penitentiary by the Committee Appointed for that Purpose by the Legislature of Maryland. Annapolis: J. Hughes, Printer, [ca. 1823].

De Tocqueville, Alexis. *On the Penitentiary System in the U.S.* 1ˢᵗ edition, 1833. Reprinted New York: Augustus M. Kelley Publishers, 1970.

{Maryland} Division of Correction Newsletter. September 1972.

Dix, Dorothea Lynde. *Remarks on Prisons and Prison Discipline in the U.S.* 2nd edition, 1845. Reprinted Montclair, N.J.: Patterson Smith, 1967.

Duncan, John Morison. *Travels through Part of the United States and Canada in 1818 and 1819.* 2 vols. Glasgow: The University Press, 1823.

Evans, Robin. *The Fabrication of Virtue: English Prison Architecture, 1750–1840.* Cambridge, U.K.: Cambridge University Press, 1982.

Farber, David. *The Age of Great Dreams: America in the 1960s.* New York: Hill & Wang, 1994.

Federal Bureau of Prisons. *Handbook of Correctional Institutional Design and Construction.* Washington, D.C.: U.S. Government Printing Office, 1949.

First Annual Report of the Committee of the Relief Association of the Maryland Penitentiary; also, the Report of the Committee of the Sabbath School Association. March 1860. Baltimore: James Lucas & Son, 1860.

Foucault, Michel. *Discipline and Punish: The Birth of the Prison.* New York: Pantheon, 1977.

Fox, Vernon. *Violence Behind Bars.* New York: Vantage Press, 1956.

Gault, Robert H. "The Parole System as a Means of Protection," *Journal of Criminal Law and Criminology,* 5 (1915).

Gettleman, Marvin. "The Maryland Penitentiary in the Age of Tocqueville, 1828–1842," *Maryland Historical Magazine,* 56 (1961): 269–90.

Gray, Francis C. *Prison Discipline in America.* London, 1848. Reprinted Montclair, N.J.: Patterson Smith, 1973.

Griffith, Thomas W. *Annals of Baltimore.* Baltimore: William Wooddy, 1824.

Hammer, Richard. *Between Life and Death.* New York: MacMillan Co., 1969.

Harley, Lewis R. *Francis Lieber: His Life and Political Philosophy.* New York: Columbia University Press, 1899.

Hartzler, Daniel. *Marylanders in the Confederacy.* Silver Spring, Md.: Family Line, 1986.

Index to the Laws of Maryland, 1800–1831.

Johnston, Norman Bruce. *Eastern State Penitentiary: Crucible of Good Intentions.* Philadelphia: Philadelphia Museum of Art, 1994.

Journal of the House of Delegates. 1820, 1822, 1825, 1826, 1834, 1836.

Journal of the Senate. 1836, 1837.

Kent, Frank R. *The Story of Maryland Politics.* Baltimore: Thomas and Evans Co., 1911.

Lambert, John R. *Arthur Pue Gorman.* Baton Rouge: Louisiana State University Press, 1953.

Latrobe, John H. B. *Picture of Baltimore, Containing a Description of All Objects of Interest in the City; and Embellished with Views of the Principal Public Buildings.* Baltimore: F. Lucas, 1832.

Laws of the State of Maryland. January–March 1890, January–April 1892.

Lewis, H. H. Walker. "Baltimore's Judicial Bombshell — Eugene O'Dunne," *American Bar Association Journal,* 56 (1970): 650-55.

Lewis, Orlando F. *The Development of American Prisons and Prison Customs, 1776–1845.* 1922. Reprinted Montclair, N.J.: Patterson Smith, 1967.

Library Catalogue — Maryland Penitentiary. Baltimore: n.d. [1937].

Livingston, Edward. *The Complete Works of Edward Livingston on Criminal Jurisprudence: Consisting of Systems of Penal Law for the State of Louisiana and for the United States of America.* 2 vols. 1833. Reprinted Montclair, N.J.: Patterson Smith, 1968.

Luxon, Norval Neil. *Niles' Weekly Register: News Magazine of the Nineteenth Century.* Baton Rouge: Louisiana State University Press, 1947.

Mannheim, Hermann, ed. *Pioneers in Criminology.* 2nd edition. Montclair, N.J.: Patterson Smith, 1972.

Marshall, Helen E. *Dorothea Dix: Forgotten Samaritan.* Chapel Hill: University of North Carolina Press, 1937.

Masur, Louis P. *Rites of Execution: Capital Punishment and the Transformation of American Culture, 1776–1865.* New York: Oxford University Press, 1989.

McEvoy, James. *Memorial to the General Assembly of Maryland by James McEvoy, Vindicatory of His Testimony Given Under Oath to the Joint Committee on the Affairs of the Penitentiary December Session 1836.* [1838].

McKelvey, Blake. *American Prisons: A History of Good Intentions.* Montclair, N.J.: Patterson Smith, 1977.

Medical Annals of Baltimore from 1608 to 1880. Baltimore: Press of Isaac Friedenwald, 1884.

Mencken, H. L. *A Mencken Chrestomathy.* New York: Alfred A. Knopf, 1949.

Mitford, Jessica. *Kind and Usual Punishment: The Prison Business.* New York: Alfred A. Knopf, 1973.

Mullen, Albert O. "Brief History of the Maryland Penitentiary from its Beginning in 1811 to the Present Time," in *Annual Report of the Maryland Penitentiary,* 1911. Baltimore, 1912. pp. 17–22.

Murphy, John. *Baltimore, the Trade Queen of the South.* 1902.

Myers, J. C. *Sketches on a Tour through the Northern and Eastern States, the Canadas and Nova Scotia.* Harrisonburg, Va.: J. H. Wartmann & Bros., 1849.

North American Review. July, 1839.

Officers of the Corporation, 1822–1883. Baltimore City Archives.

Ohlin, Lloyd, ed. *Prisoners in America: Perspectives on Our Correctional System.* Englewood Cliffs, N.J.: Prentice-Hall, Inc., 1973.

Olson, Sherry H. *Baltimore: The Building of an American City.* Baltimore: The Johns Hopkins University Press, 1980.

Papenfuse, Edward C. and Joseph M. Coale, eds. *The Hammond –Harwood House Atlas of Historical Maps of Maryland, 1608–1908.* Baltimore: The Johns Hopkins University Press, 1982.

Poppleton, T. H. *Plan of the City of Baltimore.* New York: Harrison, 1823.

Pray, Roger T. "How Did Our Prisons Get That Way?" *American Heritage,* **Vol.** 23 July/August 1987.

Proceedings of the Annual Congress of the American Prison Association. 1887–1914.

Report and accompanying documents of the House Committee appointed to examine into the affairs of the Maryland Penitentiary—Document K by the House of Delegates, July 31, 1861, and Document L by the Senate, August 1, 1861. Frederick, Md., 1861.

Reports of the Boston Prison Discipline Society, 1826–1854. 6 vols. Reprinted Montclair, N.J.: Patterson Smith, 1972.

Report of the Committee Appointed to Inspect the Situation of the Maryland Penitentiary. Annapolis: J. Hughes, Printer, 1823.

Report of Committee Appointed by Board of Directors of Maryland Penitentiary to Visit the Penitentiaries and Prisons in the City of Philadelphia and State of New York. Baltimore: Lucas & Deaver, 1828.

Report of the Committee of directors appointed to prepare plans for the new buildings to be erected in the yard of the Maryland Penitentiary. Baltimore: Lucas & Deaver, 1835.

Report of the Committee on Prison Manufactures, Maryland Penitentiary. Baltimore: Lucas & Deaver, 1842.

Report of Maryland Penitentiary Penal Commission, appointed July 24, 1912, by His Excellency Phillips Lee Goldsborough to investigate the general administration of the Maryland Penitentiary. Baltimore, 1913.

Report on Security Conditions at Maryland Penitentiary's South Wing. Baltimore: Attorney General's Office, 1984.

Report of the Select Committee on the Penitentiary to the Legislature of Maryland. Annapolis, Jeremiah Hughes, 1836.

Rothman, David. *The Discovery of Asylum: Social Order and Disorder in the New Republic.* Boston: Little, Brown, Co., 1971.

_____. *Conscience and Convenience: The Asylum and Its Alternatives in Progressive America.* Boston: Little, Brown, Co., 1980.

Rules of the State Board of Prison Control of Maryland for the Government of the Maryland Penitentiary and the House of Correction. 1921.

Rush, Benjamin. *An Enquiry into the Effects of Public Punishment upon Criminals and upon Society.* 1787.

Scharf, J. Thomas. *History of Baltimore City and County.* 1881. Reprinted Baltimore: Regional Publishing Co., 1971.

Shugg, Wallace. "The Great Escape of 'Tunnel Joe' Holmes," *Maryland Historical Magazine,* 92 (1997): 481–93.

Statements of the Board of Directors of the Maryland Penitentiary and John F. Weyler, Warden Emeritus, In Reply to the Report of Commission Maryland Penitentiary Penal System to Hon. Phillips Lee Goldsborough Governor of Maryland. Baltimore [1913].

Sullivan, Larry E. *The Prison Reform Movement: Forlorn Hope.* Boston: Twayne Publishers, 1990.

Teeters, Negley K. *The Cradle of the Penitentiary: The Walnut Street Jail at Philadelphia, 1773–1835.* Philadelphia, Sponsored by the Pennsylvania Prison Society, 1955.

Testimony Taken Before the Joint Committee of the Legislature on the Penitentiary. Annapolis, 1837.

Transactions of the National Prison Reform Congress: Held at Baltimore, Maryland, January 21–24, 1873, Being the Second Annual Meeting of the National Prison Association of the United States. Baltimore, 1873.

United States Census. 1880.

Vaux, Roberts. *Notices of the Original, and Successive Efforts to Improve the Discipline of the Prison at Philadelphia.* Philadelphia, 1826.

Walsh, Richard and William Lloyd Fox, eds. *Maryland: A History.* Annapolis: Hall of Records Commission, 1983.

Wilmer, L. Alison, J. H. Jarrett, and George W. F. Vernon. *History of the Maryland Volunteers Civil War.* Baltimore: Guggenheimer, Weil & Co., 1899.

Wines, Enoch Cobb and Theodore Dwight. *Report on the Prisons and Reformatories of the United States and Canada.* 1867. Reprinted Montclair, N.J.: Patterson Smith, 1976.

Wines, Enoch Cobb. *The State of Prisons and of Child-Saving Institutions in the United States.* 1880. Reprinted Montclair, N.J.: Patterson Smith, 1968.

Withey, Henry F. *Biographical Dictionary of American Architects (Deceased).* Los Angeles, Calif.: New Age Publishing Co., 1956.

Index

Published with the Support
of the
Joseph Meyerhoff Family Charitable Funds

Cover by James F. Brisson, Williamsville, Vermont
Book design by Gerard A. Valerio, Bookmark Studio, Annapolis, Maryland